3 4028 07066 1393
HARRIS COUNTY PUBLIC LIBRARY

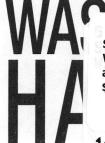

613 Sal
Saldmann, Frédéric
Wash your hands! : the dirty truth
about germs, viruses, and
$12.95   ocn230956995

1st ed.   04/01/2009

D0292759

WITHDRAWN

WASH YOUR HANDS!

THE DIRTY TRUTH ABOUT GERMS, VIRUSES, AND
EPIDEMICS—AND THE SIMPLE WAYS
TO PROTECT YOURSELF IN A
DANGEROUS WORLD

DR. FRÉDÉRIC SALDMANN

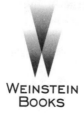

WEINSTEIN
BOOKS

© Flammarion, 2007
Translated from the French, *On s'en lave les mains*
English translation copyright © 2008 Weinstein Books LLC

All rights reserved. No part of this book may be used or reproduced in
any manner whatsoever without the written permission of the Publisher.
Printed in the United States of America. For information address
Weinstein Books, 345 Hudson Street, 13th Floor, New York, NY 10014.

ISBN: 978-1-60286-049-0

First Edition
10   9   8   7   6   5   4   3   2   1

CONTENTS

Relearning Hygiene

In the "olden days," infectious diseases wreaked havoc on a helpless populace. During the first part of the twentieth century, the discovery of germs and their role in causing infection confirmed the rules of hygiene and the notion of quarantine that our forebears had devised to fight these diseases. Antibiotics, preventive vaccinations, and other anti-infectious chemical agents seemed at first to stamp out the danger, leading us to believe that infectious diseases could be combated without much difficulty. We made great progress with surgical operations, saving more and more lives.

But every rose has its thorn. The undiscerning use of antibiotics and the neglect of basic hygienic practices, deemed obsolete in the face of infection-quashing medical miracles, have led to the growth of "super bugs," new bacterial strains each more resistant to antibiotics than the last, and the emergence of infections that are difficult to treat. Moreover, changes in eating habits and increasingly urban lifestyles, as well as the development of more-advanced technologies, have made it so that at the slightest break-down in our networks, microorganisms previously consid-ered fairly benign in pathogenic terms can multiply, spread, and cause infectious diseases, especially among the vulnerable and the elderly.

Today, we find ourselves faced with a paradox. We have at our disposal one of the most effective arsenals of cures and preventive medicines, and the most reliable facilities, and these have ameliorated our lifestyles and surroundings, yet we're confronted by fearsome microorganisms and often-deadly infectious diseases. We must take the time to relearn all the rules of hygiene, old and new alike, for they will help limit contamination and infection from germs on and around us. The rules of hygiene passed down to us by our elders, in combination with those tailored to new, contem-porary situations, will help us live longer, better lives, es-pecially in cases where treatments do not yet exist or are no longer effective.

Fabien Squinazi, M.D.
Director, Laboratory of Hygiene of the City of Paris

INTRODUCTION

Danger breeds best on too much confidence.
—PIERRE CORNEILLE

When I was a child, my mother always told me, "An ounce of prevention is worth a pound of cure." Much later, as a doctor, I finally understood how right she was. When medicine opened its secrets to me, I became aware of the damage that lack of information can do to the body. Imagine a smoker who doesn't know how dangerous tobacco is: That person would be risking his or her health without having made the choice to do so. Full knowledge of the health hazards involved in a given act is essential to the prevention of illness.

That's why I decided, a few years ago, to devote my energy to developing prevention and awareness programs at the individual and group levels. No easy task, for doctors usually find themselves in the same position as dentists: patients seek them out only when suffering from toothache, when an earlier checkup might have averted the problem.

As a number of serious diseases betray few or no apparent symptoms, patients often don't feel the need for regular checkups, when in fact such visits could make all the difference.

Cardiology, my first area of study, provides a perfect illustration. It takes a dozen years or so for a coronary artery to get clogged up and cause a heart attack. But a number of risk factors, such as excess weight, lack of exercise, stress, hypertension, high cholesterol, and high blood sugar can accelerate the process. For a patient to become aware of these factors, spot their own symptoms in time, and take action to modify his or her habits amounts to a great victory for the doctor as well as the patient.

Thanks to simple preventive measures, starting with a healthy diet, the heart attack victim who might have spent his or her days wheezing from chair to bed can not only avoid further cardiovascular mishap, but also get back into shape and enjoy life to the fullest. Hippocrates highlighted this link centuries before modern medicine when he said, "Let food be thy medicine, and let thy medicine be food."

Ten years ago, when I wrote *Omega-3*, I happened upon a striking fact: Eskimos and Japanese people, who take in omega-3 fatty acids daily thanks to a diet rich in fish, have the lowest myocardial infarction rates on the planet. It was clear that omega-3 fatty acids play an undeniable part in protecting the body's cardiovascular system—and the taking of omega-3 supplements became a trend. Still, the regular consumption of foods high in omega-3s is not enough for a healthy diet, which is above all balanced, varied, and free of toxins and microbial contamination. A healthy diet is just one of the habits that constitute proper hygiene. Just what does good hygiene consist of, anyway?

From that moment on, I worked long and hard on the rules of hygiene: the habits that, taken together, form our best preventive tool kit. In writing *The New Dietary Dangers* (Ramsay, 1997) around the time of the "mad cow" scare, I offered a guide to help people better protect themselves against emerging dangers. Faced with the news of dioxin contamination and other pollutants, as well as repeated outbreaks of listeriosis and Creutzfeldt-Jakob disease, many people no longer knew what to do. Most important to impress upon everyone was the necessity of hand washing. I cited a British study, since referenced many times in the media, exposing the presence of fourteen different urine traces in a bowl of peanuts at a pub. The source was obvious: Customers were sticking their hands in the bowls without having washed them before leaving the bathroom. This astonishing discovery led me to the realization not only of the frequency of certain dangers but also the simple measures that can be taken to avoid them.

Unfortunately, new menaces have appeared since the turn of the century, and it's more than likely we will undergo major crises in the years to come. The first warning signs are showing up in cases of avian flu. This is only the beginning. Viral diseases are surfacing all the time, with significant pandemics in the offing. Whether because of the ease and frequency of travel, global warming, or population growth, scientists have warned for years that the stage is being set for the advent of some particularly problematic health conditions.

Denying this fact would be as futile as getting overly alarmed by it. In order to combat the coming crises, we will need to learn and relearn the rules of hygiene, which are all too easily neglected in modern life. While dangers specific to our times do exist, so do the measures to prevent them.

This book takes stock of which hygienic habits are truly useful and which are less so, in order to provide the keys to effective prevention—still our best defense in the years to come.

PART I

THE BASICS

In today's world, everything moves faster than before. Increased global trade, ever-greater numbers of travelers, immigrants moving farther than ever before, a constantly growing population: the world is, in effect, accelerating. This gives rise to new dangers in our daily lives, especially if, for lack of time or information, we come to neglect the fundamentals of hygiene, which can spare us many an inconvenience.

The Deadly Handshake

I've been known to refuse to shake someone's hand,
but less from conviction than from reasons of hygiene.
—Pierre Drachline

In one of his short stories, "The Man Who Would Not
Shake Hands," Stephen King introduces readers to a
Londoner who has just won a game of poker: a certain Mr.
Brower, who was put under a curse while in Bombay. To
congratulate him, his challenger shakes his hand, starts
screaming at the top of his lungs, tries to flee, and then dies
violently of a heart attack.

What if this horror story bore some relation to reality?

Shaking the hand of someone who's just landed at
O'Hare with cholera can certainly infect you—not because
the germs pass through the skin, but because we often
bring our hands to our mouths. We cover our mouths when
coughing or yawning, we pick at bits of food between our
teeth with toothpicks, and we eat with our fingers.

Hands can carry many germs. Just imagine, for a moment, someone coughing. That someone brings a hand

to his or her mouth out of consideration for those nearby. Admittedly a wise precaution, but one that will in fact spray millions of germs contained in tiny droplets of saliva across that person's palm. If that person should shake your hand a minute later, the germs would be transmitted to your hand, and then from your hand to your mouth.

In practice, hands are privileged vectors for two types of germs. The first comes from the respiratory system, a flu virus or a rhinovirus. Studies have shown that 70 percent of people with a cold have, on their hands, the very bacteria that are to blame for it. The second and clearly more dangerous type of germ comes from the digestive tract: cholera vibrio, Staphylococcus, Salmonella, and various dysentery-causing Shigellae can be found on our hands by way of fecal matter. These can cause serious diarrhea and even, in the case of certain bacteria like *Helicobacter pylori*, gastric ulcers. Just a few germs are enough: once swallowed, the warm and humid conditions of the digestive tract allow them to multiply until they trigger severe problems.

How long a germ can survive on the hands depends on its type. Those from the respiratory tract do not have a long life span at all, and if any transmission occurs, it generally takes place immediately. Those from the digestive tract, on the other hand, can survive several hours, unless the carrier washes his or her hands properly, an essential habit. If a carrier of cholera vibrio forgets to do so upon leaving the bathroom, he or she risks passing it on to someone else with as little as a simple handshake, or by serving food or touching a surface another person might touch. Cholera is a particularly illuminating example: this illness has an incubation period of up to three weeks, during which there are no symptoms, and the infected subject may infect countless others before becoming aware that he or she is sick. Each subject in turn has the potential to unknowingly produce an outbreak of cholera, with its life threatening symptoms of diarrhea, dehydration, and fever, likely to lead victims straight to the ICU unit at the nearest hospital.

Fecal Bacteria in the Mouth? After a Mere Handshake?

If you shake hands with someone who's just come from the bathroom without washing his or her hands, there is a one in three chance of getting germs from that person's feces in your mouth within two hours. Don't believe me?

In order to precisely evaluate the extent of bacterial transmission when two people shake hands, I conducted two studies with Dr. Fabien Squinazi, director of the Laboratory of Hygiene of the City of Paris, in December 2006 and January 2007. The goal in each was the same: to measure the number of germs present on people who had shaken hands with those who carried fecal bacteria on their hands after going to the bathroom. The carriers themselves could have been contaminated, either by not washing their own hands, or by the intermediary of a dirty doorknob.

The tests, conducted on fifteen people, revealed that no less than eleven of them (or 73 percent, approximately three out of four people), had ended up with germs on their hands. Ten were carriers of the fecal bacteria E. coli, and the other five of *Tatumella ptyseos*.

Faced with results of such surprising proportions, we ran the same study again in January 2007, on eighteen individuals. This time, nine of them (or 50 percent, the equivalent of one out of two people) received fecal germs, but of greater variety. We identified, in effect, two cases of *Serratia plymuthica*, two cases of *Citrobacter freundii*, one of *Proteus penneri*, one of *Erwinia*, one of *Escherichia coli*, and two combining E. coli and *S. plymuthica*. We decided to go even farther and take samples from the lips two hours after contact with the carrier. In the intervening time, participants in the study were offered coffee and snacks.

The first important observation was that during this interval, all test subjects brought their hands to their mouths several times, whether to eat or to cover their mouths when coughing or yawning. The second: these hand movements definitely led to contamination. In fact, three carriers showed traces of contamination on their lips: two by *Serratia plymuthica*, and one by E. coli in combination with *S. plymuthica*. Samples taken from the others' lips showed five cases of transmission: three for E. coli, one for *S. plymuthica*, and one for *Erwinia*. In total, seven out of eighteen people showed evidence of contamination on their lips—in other words, a shocking 39 percent, or one in three people!

The findings of these two experiments brook no appeal: An individual carrying fecal bacteria on his or her hands—the gastroenteritis or stomach flu virus, for example—can contaminate between 50 and 73 percent of the people he or she shakes hands with. In a third of the cases, fecal contamination then spreads to the lips when the hands are brought to the mouth. This explains why diseases like gastroenteritis, which is spread by manual contact, can affect so many people in such a short time.

In conclusion, the diffusion of fecal germs is much more sizable than one might imagine. Moreover, other studies have all reached similar conclusions.

Proven Risks

If, today, the connection between manual hygiene and the onset of illness is no longer in doubt, this hasn't always been the case, as is shown by the story of the Hungarian physician Ignace Semmelweiss. Semmelweiss was the first to establish, in 1848, the relation between lack of hand washing and the extremely high death rate among newborns due to puerperal fever. He tried to impose the washing of hands and changing of clothes on medical workers entering the workplace, but to no avail. Worse yet, his newfangled ideas got him banished from Vienna to Pest (today part of Budapest), where he suffered a nervous breakdown, dying shortly thereafter in a Viennese asylum.

Science has since vindicated him, and scientists continue to show great interest in hands as vectors of infection as they try to learn more about disease. Recent studies have been conducted in the States to determine the serious risks connected to improper manual hygiene. One University of Colorado study in particular has highlighted the significant role hands play in spreading germs. Four hundred students living on campus were split into two groups. For the first group, dispensers with hand-washing solution were installed everywhere: the cafeteria, bedrooms, bathrooms, etc. For the second group, housed in a separate building, no such equipment or incentive to wash one's hands was put in place. The experiment lasted six months and was positively illuminating. Researchers noted 20 percent fewer cases of illness, especially respiratory, in the first group relative to the second, and 43 percent fewer absences from class.

Other studies conducted on a hundred students in Maryland high schools revealed an interesting behavioral aspect to manual hygiene. When students found themselves alone in bathrooms, 45 percent "forgot" to wash their hands. But in the presence of their peers, only 9 percent failed to wash. We can well believe the same thing goes on in public places. Other people's gazes keep us from our own blameworthy negligence by obliging us to wash our hands, whereas, alone, we might not necessarily do it. Yet, as the

University of Colorado study showed, this simple act of personal hygiene protects the individual from contracting certain illnesses in a very measurable way.

A Habit Up for Reappraisal

Given the risks just outlined, I cannot keep myself from a moment's pity for all those politicians who have to shake thousands of hands at events, rallies, or fairs, where they must also politely nibble on everything thrust at them. An episode from the second season of the TV series *24* portrays an attempt on the life of the American president via a toxic substance a terrorist conceals in the palm of her hand. By shaking the president's hand at a meeting, she contaminates him and he crumples to the ground a few hours later.

In France and much of the West, we are in the habit of shaking hands all the time. The custom originated with the early Christians, who saw the handshake as a sign of sharing. The gesture seems natural, but it is far from shared by the rest of the world. A handshake is not a universal habit; Asians prefer to put their hands together and offer a slight bow.

Whatever the handshake is meant to represent, it is difficult to refuse an extended hand in our culture. *Very* difficult, in fact. Instead of being overlooked, the refusal of a handshake will likely constitute a veritable offense: the person whose hand was declined may have a hard time forgiving you. In much the same way, it would be unthinkable, whether for reasons of politeness or mere practicality, to run and wash your hands after shaking those of your friends. What then, are we to do? Here's some advice applicable to everyday use.

For starters, we might teach our children another way to greet people, since young children are forever bringing their hands to their mouths. Without going so far as to limit them to curtseys and bows, why not instill in them the habit of saying hello with a simple, friendly wave? They will quickly catch on that handshakes are for grownups.

Next, it's better to place your hand at a slight distance in front of your mouth when coughing or yawning. This reduces the risk of spreading germs. In addition, wash your hands thoroughly with soap before and after using a toothpick.

If washing your hands before eating or snacking proves impossible, avoid touching food directly by picking it up with a napkin or some other disposable wrapper. Ideally, one should always carry disposable Handi Wipes or Wet-Nap towels to disinfect one's hands. These are readily available at most drugstores.

Finally, we can try to limit the handshakes we give and receive without offending the people around us. A simple look can say more than an outstretched hand. To reduce the number of possible occasions for a handshake, try not to take the initiative when meeting someone you know. A warm smile, a small pat on the shoulder, or a gesture of welcome with the arms can largely compensate for a hand-shake. Discriminating use of this gesture is also a way to restore all its symbolic value. Replacing it with a kiss on the cheek is also possible, except in certain cases: people with active colds, flus, herpes simplex, or digestive infections should refuse to kiss or be kissed, if only out of a sense of civic responsibility to others.

Tips for Optimal Hand Washing

Hand washing is indispensable. But we must go even far-ther by taking an interest in how most effectively to rid the hands of undesirable germs. Hand washing, when per-formed with care, includes the cuticles and spaces between fingers, and is followed by a generous rinsing. Beware: if these steps aren't followed by a full and complete drying, their very usefulness can be turned against them. Any resid-ual moisture on the skin or between fingers promotes bac-terial proliferation. Tests have shown that moist hands transmit five hundred times as many germs as dry ones.*

Drying not only serves to get rid of water from rinsing, but also helps wipe away the products of hand washing as well as remaining grime and flakes of skin (cutaneous squama). Ultimately, the drying process helps reduce the

---

*From a study cited in *Cleaning & Maintenance Management* maga-zine, December 2001.

number of bacteria present on the skin. That is why I make a point of insisting on this often neglected step. In a survey conducted on 7,700 users of public bathrooms in Germany, France, Holland, and Switzerland by the European Association for the Promotion of Hand Hygiene, 34 percent* did not bother drying their hands. Hardly surprising—how many of us have been satisfied with a quick shake over the sink instead of a careful drying? Reasons cited usually include lack of time and an ignorance of the benefits of this act. The convenience of the means of drying made available, in terms of comfort, efficacy, and swiftness, also plays its part. Different studies have tried to find the best hand-drying solutions.

Hygienic Hand Drying

Any means of hand drying must prove to be hygienically beyond reproach, lest the drying undo the benefits of washing and reduce hands to a state even less microbiologically desirable. The following should be avoided in public as a rule:

- Shared towels of any fabric, such as hand towels, which remain damp and dirty, recontaminating hands during drying

---

*"Dirty Hands." *Bulletin of the European Association for the Promotion of Hand Hygiene* (April 1996): 156–7.

- Warm-air hand dryers. Wet hands combined with warm air provide ideal conditions for the growth of bacteria.

A study carried out by Dr. Georges Ducel and others from Laboratory of Hygiene at the Cantonal University Hospital of Geneva, published in the October 1998 issue of *Techniques hospitalières* [Hospital Technology] shows that the number of germs present on the skin of people who washed their hands and then dried them with a warm-air dryer was greater than that present on the skin before washing. By using this kind of device, one actually collects germs from the hands of other users as well as the air itself, because germs are drawn by the airflow into the machine, where they then multiply in the heat and humidity.

To illustrate this phenomenon, a germ count was performed on the surface of the hands—an area of about 3.7 square inches—on two groups of subjects. The first dried their hands with paper towels and clocked in at an average of about 137 germs before washing, 117 after washing, and 47 after drying and wiping. The second group dried their hands with a warm-air dryer and averaged 127 before washing, 110 after, and 206 after drying. The numbers speak for themselves. Moreover, hot air often dries out the skin.

I recommend, therefore, the use of textile towels, whether in a continuous roll or in a single-use dispenser. The first allows each user to wipe his or her hands on a segment of clean cloth that is automatically wound back into the machine.

According to the aforementioned study by Dr. Ducel, this
method reduces the number of germs on the skin by half
from after washing to the end of drying. There is nothing
anecdotal about the evidence.

Paper towels are an equally sanitary solution, but their
use necessitates a trash receptacle. They can also quickly
prove more costly than the reusable, continuous cloth solution mentioned above.

The importance of washing—and drying!—one's hands
cannot be stressed enough. The practice of this simple act
on a daily basis goes a long way toward the prevention of
microbial contamination.

Intestinal Hygiene

There are only two things a child will share willingly:
communicable diseases and his mother's age.
—BENJAMIN SPOCK

We live in what seems an increasingly antiseptic world.
It seems inconceivable that intestinal parasites might
still thrive at the heart of our perfect, immaculate universe.
This is, however, the case. Although their frequency has
been, on the whole, falling since the 1960s, they have in
the last few years made a comeback. How can this phenomenon be explained?

Oft-cited is the ease of travel and air transport, which
permits parasites to roam the planet in every direction, but
this alone does not account for the change. It is, above all,
the slide in standards of daily hygiene that must be held
responsible. We have forgotten certain simple rules that
have long proved their effectiveness.

Life in any community favors close and frequent contact, particularly among children, and thereby the spread

of parasites. Increased enrollment in schools and the proliferation of day-care centers, to name but two examples,
entail new rules of hygiene, even as most former hygienic
practices remain relevant against the various intestinal
parasites discussed here. A later chapter in the section on
foods will be devoted entirely to a single parasite and its
preferred habitat—tapeworms found in beef—while bacterial afflictions will be covered in the chapter titled
"Emerging Vectors of Disease."

The Pinworm Pest

Intestinal pinworms, members of the *Oxyuridae* family, are
quite common, if rarely discussed, no doubt because the
symptoms accompanying them—recurrent anal itching,
often at night—inspire a certain reticence among affected
subjects.

The culprit is usually *Enterobius vermicularis*, which
measures, on average, just under half an inch in length.
This worm and its ilk thrive in a very specific part of the
digestive tract: the ileum and the cecum, which constitute
the beginning of the large intestine. At night, the females
migrate toward the anus to lay eggs, which are known for
their powers of survival and their high infectious potential.
The eggs can then be dispersed on underwear, sheets, and
even on the ground.

People contaminate themselves by ingesting the eggs unknowingly. Once in the intestine, these eggs hatch larvae that reach maturity three weeks later. Children are the first to be affected, often followed by those who spend their time around them.

Any difficulty in diagnosing the presence of pinworms resides in the fact that parasitological exams often come back negative. It is not easy to find adult worms in stool samples. The most effective diagnostic technique consists of applying a ribbon of Scotch tape to the anus in the morning and sending it to a lab for analysis after a few hours. As soon as the presence of pinworms has been confirmed, a simple treatment can bring the infestation to an end. The medication ointment is often prescribed in two cycles, with a fifteen-day interval between, to prevent any possible recurrence.

As with many diseases, the best solution for pinworm infestation remains prevention. The most effective means is to wash one's hands as often as necessary, especially upon waking in the morning, before leaving the bathroom, and before every meal. Fingernails should be kept clean and clipped. Parents should be aware that neglect on the part of schools in keeping up the soap supply in bathrooms can help pinworms spread. It is surprising to see entire families who continue to suffer from pinworms—forced to undergo regular treatment—when respecting simple rules of hygiene would rid them of their undesirable guests.

Giardiasis

Originally, this parasite was only found in tropical areas, but now it is frequently encountered in North America and, in Europe especially, in nurseries and small collectives.

Unlike pinworms, giardias develop in the small intestine. They sometimes cause diarrhea and, less frequently, greasy stools and weight loss. In some cases, the infected subject betrays no symptoms. Examination of the stools results in diagnosis and the prescription of nitroimidazole-based medications. In order to avoid reinfection, it is essential to extend the treatment to the subject's circle of family and friends.

Humans become infected by ingesting cysts present in water, raw foods, or on dirty hands, the last of which can easily pass cysts on to friends and loved ones. Some parts of the world are more at risk than others: travelers returning from the Caribbean or northern Africa, for example, may have contracted the parasite while there. Children are frequently affected after stays in these regions, but the parasite can also be transmitted at home, via foods from the far-flung corners of the world. All the more reason to wash foods carefully, to peel fruits and vegetables or cook them thoroughly, and always to keep raw foods separate from cooked foods in the refrigerator.

Generally speaking, travelers must bear in mind a few basic rules of hygiene. Getting just a glimpse of some commercial kitchens is enough to make one realize that tap water in one- and five-star hotels alike comes from a single public source. In order to avoid disagreeable surprises, opt for dishes cooked at more than 160 degrees Fahrenheit, as these are without great risk, especially when served piping hot. Peel all fruit with care, including tomatoes eaten uncooked, and always go for bottled drinks.

Amoebas

Entamoeba histolytica thrive primarily in the liver, but can be found in the intestine as well. In certain cases, they can cause dysentery, abscesses of the intestinal wall, and infectious metastases toward other organs. The colon is the first to be affected; amoebas then colonize the liver, causing abscesses that can sometimes be quite sizable.

Contamination occurs by means of *Entamoeba histolytica* cysts. Highly resistant—indeed, capable of surviving fifteen days in water at any temperature between 32 and 77 degrees Fahrenheit—they can be found on the surfaces of foods. When these foods are consumed, the cysts transform into metacystic amoebas in their new host.

Foods are a rather everyday mode of transmission. As a result, amoebiasis is a widespread type of parasitosis. Ten percent of the world's population are currently contaminated—a considerable number.* Although this disease affects people everywhere, the number of infected subjects

—————
*D. A. Brockner, "Amœbiasis," *Clinical Microbiology Review* (October 1992): 356–69.

in tropical regions is proportionally far greater than elsewhere, where most cases are brought by travelers. Therefore, keep the problem of amoebas in mind when you return from travels abroad.

Atypical symptoms are likely to betray the company of amoebas: unexplained fatigue, minor weight loss, temporary bowel trouble. What must be stressed is that people who look healthy regularly spread the parasites without knowing it. The presence of parasites often goes unnoticed, and infected subjects give no thought to it. A parasitological examination of stool samples is required for diagnosis. Effective treatments do exist. Get an exam at the slightest cause for concern, and you'll quickly track down possible amebiasis and prevent serious complications.

Ticks, Lice, and Fleas:
Carriers of Many a Disease

Between dog and master is but the hop of a flea.
—JULES RENARD

L ice, fleas, and ticks proliferate in the world around us, passing easily from host to host. There has been a fresh upsurge in such parasite cases, which commonly involve bothersome but benign symptoms well known to the public: rashes and itching, among them.

Less well known is that a simple tick bite can cause a condition far more serious than a mere itch. In fact, in certain countries, these creatures are carriers of diseases potentially deadly to human beings.

Lyme Disease

Lyme disease was first observed in the 1970s, in a small Connecticut town that, by lending the illness its name, entered into the annals of medicine without any corresponding gain to its attractiveness as a tourist destination.

There is nothing attractive about the disease. The culprit is a spirochete of the genus *Borrelia*, equipped with seven flagella that keep it in a state of constant rotation. There are three different species, each inducing its own set of symptoms, which explains variations in the disease from one country to another.

Lyme disease is well known today, and is considered a professional hazard for forest workers. Leisure activities like camping and off-road biking put one at risk. Whether you're a cyclist or a lumberjack, being in the woods—especially during high season, from spring through fall—exposes you to deer ticks. These creatures are veritable reservoirs of *Borrelia*, which they transmit to humans via bites.

After the bite, the disease unfolds in three stages. The first, called Lipschütz's *erythema chronicum migrans*, shows up as a redness around the bite itself. Ringlike skin lesions may soon follow or can take as long as a month or more to appear. In most cases, the legs and thighs are affected, and to a lesser extent, the face and scalp as well.

The lesion is characterized by a red macule or papule—a reddened patch of skin that can be either level or raised—of up to four inches. It does not itch. The infected subject may experience headaches, a low fever, and glandular swelling in the region of the initial lesion. Most often, these flulike symptoms will go away in four to five weeks, leaving no trace.

The problem is that the underlying disease itself does

not go away. As a general rule, the secondary or late stage occurs in the months or even years following the bite. Severe chronic joint pain often develops, frequently involving the knees. The pain occurs in attacks and is migratory: sometimes only a single joint is affected, and at other times, several at once. The symptoms worsen with each attack. In untreated cases, the infection spreads to the heart and nervous system. Cardiac complications arise, sometimes in the form of myocarditis (inflammation of the heart muscle) or pericarditis (inflammation of the sac surrounding the heart). Myocarditis can involve cardiac conduction problems that necessitate emergency hospitalization because of the heightened risk of heart attack and heart failure. Both conditions can cause marked shortness of breath, even during moderate activity.

Nervous-system manifestations of the infection can affect the cranial and especially facial nerves, and can even result in meningitis.

In the third stage of untreated disease, long after the initial tick bite has been forgotten, even more serious troubles arise, such as Pick-Herxheimer's disease, also known as Taylor's disease (*acrodermatitis chronica atrophicans*), a syndrome common in Europe that manifests itself as progressive thinning of the skin, such that nerves are eventually visible through it. In rare cases, dementia has been recorded.

Considering these serious complications, it's clear that consulting a physician at the slightest possibility of having been bitten, or if you're experiencing cardiac, neurological, or joint disorders of mysterious origin, is a must. The disease can be detected by the ELISA (enzyme-linked immunoabsorbent assay) blood test and confirmed by the Western blot test, which uses antibody labeling. Treatment consists of antibiotics, which have, thus far, proved effective.

At the time of writing there is unfortunately no effective means of preventing the disease other than avoiding places where ticks are found and wearing protective clothing. No effective vaccine is currently available, and ticks are very resistant to insecticides. Certain measures must be taken after a tick bite. The tick must be removed as soon as possible, taking care not to break the tick's rostrum, the mouthparts embedded in the skin. It is not necessarily essential to start a prophylactic antibiotic regimen afterward, as not all ticks are infectious. However, specialists systematically recommend that all pregnant women do so to avoid infecting the fetus.

Lyme disease is present on all continents and can remain dormant for a long time. Doctors and patients should keep the disease in mind as a possibility when diagnosing joint pain that arises years after an apparently harmless bite.

Chagas' Disease

This lesser-known illness, concentrated in South America, affects 18 million people the world over. According to an article by Anis Rassi Jr., M.D., and Sérgio G. Rassi, M.D., in *Circulation*, each year it strikes 300,000 more people, killing 21,000 of them. The reason for the spread of the disease is the common "kissing bug."

The guilty party is a trypanosome known as *Trypanosoma cruzi*, carried by hematophagous, or bloodsucking, insects that have a two-year life-span. Their bite is not painful and usually occurs while the victim is asleep. Though the subject remains asleep and unaware, the trypanosomes are already at work, soon to be found in the blood, infecting the heart, muscles, and nervous system. The incubation period is generally one to two weeks, during which a chagoma, or small skin nodule, sometimes appears at the site of the bite.

Next, more serious symptoms appear: a high fever involving the glands and swelling of the liver and spleen. Complications may include congestive heart failure.

Physicians diagnose the disease with a blood test, using the "thick drop" technique. Antibiotics are used to treat the acute phase, but are not helpful in chronic cases left untreated.

Effective preventive measures are therefore in everyone's best interest. These consist of making one's living quarters cleaner and healthier—eliminating cracks and fissures, crumbling walls, or thatched roofs well-loved by kissing bugs. Last but not least, remain watchful when traveling and sleeping in less-than-sanitary conditions, and don't hesitate to see a doctor upon your return if you think you may have been exposed.

Lice: Allies of Illness

Every parent knows that lice cause skin lesions, especially on the scalp, but how many know that these invasive critters can also cause many diseases, like exanthematous or epidemic typhus, or relapsing fever? A thorough accounting of the issue would no doubt be useful, all the more so since many social settings have seen a renewed upsurge in lice—especially head lice.

You guessed it—there is more than one kind of louse:

- body louse (*Pediculus humanus corporis*)—often found in folds of clothing
- head louse (*Pediculus humanus capitis*)—lays its eggs (the infamous nits) at the roots of hair
- pubic louse (*Phthirus pubis*)—commonly called crabs, lives in pubic hair

Whatever the kind in question, transmission can be direct or indirect. The subject can infect others through bodily contact—on the playground during recess, at an after-school sport or, in the case of pubic lice, during sexual relations. In other cases, lice are spread through borrowed hats and combs, shared sheets, and toilet seats. School is one of the most frequent sites for transmission.

There is no cause for alarm in the majority of cases: lice betray their presence with minor skin lesions and persistent itching—an annoyance, to be sure, but not really dangerous in themselves. They can often be diagnosed with the naked eye: flat white nits are easily seen on the scalp, while body lice show up as small moving black dots. A magnifying glass is best for spotting pubic lice.

Once their presence is confirmed, localized external treatments should be started immediately. Many effective products are available over the counter, but beware: the safety of some of these is disputed, especially in the case of products for children. Pregnant women are advised not to use powder treatments, which may be toxic. Don't hesitate to ask your pharmacist for advice on selecting the product best suited to your needs.

No matter what product you settle on, no treatment will be fully effective unless it is accompanied by hygienic measures, which greatly reduce the chance of indirect transmission. When a household is colonized by lice, it is essential to clean toys, brushes, and combs thoroughly to avoid further outbreaks. The same goes for sheets, blankets, and clothes, which should be washed in water at temperatures of at least 140 degrees Fahrenheit.

To those who find such measures a bit excessive, let it be said that lice are not to be taken lightly. Although cases of lice-borne diseases have noticeably declined, they persist in remote or isolated areas of the world. Such places are beginning to draw tourists and volunteer workers. Thanks to transportation today, an isolated village that is a hotbed of infection is but a few hours by plane from up-to-date medical attention. Encouraging these regions to put sanitary policies in place remains a crucial campaign in the fight against epidemics.

Louse-borne relapsing fever has long been officially recognized. The agent responsible is a virus named *Borrelia recurrentis*, for which body lice and bedbugs are vectors, or carriers. People often infect themselves by crushing the insects, thus unwittingly freeing the virus, which enters the body and causes the disease. It presents as a high fever, difficult digestion, and swelling of the spleen. Luckily, effective antibiotic treatments exist today, but in the past, relapsing fever was the cause of major epidemics, the last of which occurred in 1940 and affected 10 million people. Today, such epidemics are confined to countries like Ethiopia, Somalia, and Sudan, and are subsiding.

Epidemic typhus, also carried by body lice, is disappearing from the world as well: according to the World Health Organization, there were only 7,500 cases in 1980. Also treatable with antibiotics, its symptoms are a high fever accompanied by skin marks. The last known pockets of disease were traced to Ethiopia and the mountainous regions of South America. Like embers capable of reigniting a fire, these pockets of disease put entire countries at risk. Propagation occurs with surprising rapidity and quickly leads to serious situations. In order to keep outbreaks from occurring, it behooves us to remain vigilant about cleanliness.

Fleas

These tiny insects, measuring an eighth of an inch and possessing three pairs of legs, are also vectors of disease, including the one that has had the greatest impact on humankind: bubonic plague. A single bite from a tainted flea is enough to infect a human being.

Luckily, the plague has almost disappeared: only 36,876 cases were reported over the last few years in the twenty-four countries of Asia, Africa, and South America where infectious pockets still exist. This is far from the 25 million deaths in Europe alone during the fourteenth century.

The most common symptoms of flea bites are papular skin lesions with accompanying pruritus, or itching. However, in certain tropical regions (parts of Africa, the Caribbean, and the Seychelles), sand fleas, or chiggers (the chigoe flea, or *Tunga penetrans*) can cause more serious disorders. They are capable of burrowing deep into the skin, where they lay their eggs. Five days later, pea-size nodules appear beneath the skin, often causing acute inflammation. These fleas make their homes in the sand, so prevention consists quite simply of not going barefoot in their habitat.

Mycoses All Over

Mushrooms grow in moist places. That's why they take the shape of an umbrella.

—ALPHONSE ALLAIS

The word *mycosis* refers to a condition caused by the presence of parasitic fungi. These exist in great number. Some are superficial (cutaneous) and affect skin, nails, or mucous membranes, while others are systemic, like aspergillus, which affects the lungs.

They all have one thing in common: the frequency of related cases has skyrocketed in the last few years. This upsurge can be explained by various factors, as we shall see. In any case, combating fungi requires specific measures in addition to the ordinary rules of hygiene.

Some Superficial Mycoses

The most common of the superficial mycoses is intertrigo, otherwise known as athlete's foot. It causes an inflammation of moist body folds. Feet are not the only affected part:

Folds beneath the breasts and between buttocks or fi[...] can also be affected. The fungus, which proliferates on skin squamae (scales) left on damp surfaces such as those at poolsides, is easily transmitted to those walking barefoot. Failure to dry the body thoroughly with a clean towel further encourages fungal growth. Dampness in general promotes fungal growth, as do shoes and synthetic fabrics. Sometimes the resulting itchy rash oozes and becomes infected. Overweight individuals and diabetics are more prone to this kind of infection.

Another mycosis, pityriasis versicolor, causes pink or pale spots on the skin after exposure to sun. Recurrence is common, even after treatment. Still another, tinea circinata, or ringworm, a round, itchy skin lesion, is found on people who live in close contact with animals. Oral thrush is the best known of candidiases, or yeast infections, that affect the digestive tract. It manifests itself as white patches against a red, erythematic, or inflamed, tongue and oral cavity. Its close cousin, genital candidiasis, often called vaginal yeast, can be exacerbated by certain factors: oral contraceptives, antibiotic treatments, or the existence of diabetes.

Fungi can also lodge under fingernails, as is the case with mycotic perionyxis and onychomycosis. Working with one's hands plunged into moist environments promotes the appearance of such complaints. The nails grow yellowish and pus may ooze from them. Last in this rather unappetizing survey is tinea capitis, or ringworm of the scalp, which shows up as hairless patches—these too are due to fungi.

The rise in fungal afflictions can first be explained by the increasing numbers of people susceptible to them: diabetics, the elderly, and AIDS patients. Second, to the availability of both locally applied antiseptic treatments and repeated rounds of antibiotics, which disrupt the body's normal microbial ecology. There exists, on the skin and mucous membranes, a balance among bacteria and fungi. When these chemical treatments suddenly turn up, they upset the fragile equilibrium, giving formerly unimportant microorganisms an opportunity to develop. Certain fungi require but a tiny helping hand to take over and proliferate, leading to disease.

Medical progress has itself given rise to pathogens. Among women, for example, oral contraceptives increase the risk of mycoses by disturbing natural mechanisms, and thereby providing a breeding ground for yeast.

Lack of proper hygiene also contributes. The dirty puddles and footbaths of public pools breed mycoses. The other factors we've mentioned may be difficult to control, but attention to hygiene is well within everyone's reach. Taking a shower before and after a swim in the pool and drying off well are simple, sanitary acts, as is avoiding the lending or borrowing of socks, combs, and bathrobes. These few elementary measures allow us to greatly reduce the chance of contracting a cutaneous mycosis such as ringworm or athlete's foot—what about the systemic ones?

Systemic, But Not Systematic

Systemic mycoses have also seen a recent recrudescence, which may be explained in part by the rising number of immunodepressed patients—that is, people whose immune systems are compromised, leaving them more vulnerable to fungi capable of attacking their organs.

Among systemic afflictions, aspergillosis is the most common. Caused by aspergillus, a frequently occurring filamentous mold often found on organic remains, this disease has traits typical of its category. Dust suspended in the air can contain mold spores, which, when inhaled, can be life threatening, especially among weakened patients.

Indeed, this fungus knows how to turn situations to its advantage in finding itself a home. Invasive pulmonary aspergillosis is, for example, widespread among patients associated with hospitals undergoing renovations that raise dust. In addition, patients already hospitalized often have more fragile immune defenses. They may also have been victims of prior pulmonary afflictions that have left cavities, as from tuberculosis, in which aspergillus may lodge. These weakened patients are, in fact, breeding grounds for fungal expansion. Their heightened susceptibility shows the degree to which air quality control is essential for good health. From this perspective, it goes without saying that the maintenance of ventilation systems is fundamental, especially in a hospital setting.

Attack of the Dust Mites

There are timid people who look under their beds, and
timid people who don't dare look under their beds.
—JULES RENARD

D o dust mites really need an introduction? If one considers the number of articles published on them in the mainstream press, the countless reports that have been devoted to them, and the mattresses and pillows that purport to combat them, it seems redundant. Not so, however—in reality, dust mite allergies are more and more common, and are the cause of as many pathologies among children as among adults. Which proves, despite the public awareness campaigns, that much remains to be learned where prevention is concerned. Besides, how well do we really know dust mites? Do we really have an idea of the dangers they represent?

Stars of the Allergy World

Beneath a microscope, the dust mite can be seen to have a rounded abdomen and four pairs of hairy legs equipped with hooks or suckers. They are found in household dust, and proliferate in less frequently visited dwellings like vacation or country homes. They have an average life-span of three months, during which females can lay up to two hundred eggs, according to the Food and Agriculture Organization of the United Nations. Feeding on human squamae—or sloughed-off skin cells—and animal dander, as well as other organic debris, they love high temperatures and humidity, which encourage their reproduction.

It is not the creatures themselves that are harmful, but rather their excrement, which contains particularly powerful allergens. The threshold beyond which allergy attacks are triggered is related to several parameters. If a person has suffered from allergies to dust mites in the past, the allergen concentration necessary to set off another attack is lower. An average rate of one hundred mites per pound of dust may suffice. Heredity also plays its part: if one or both parents is allergic, a child runs a higher-than-average risk of being allergic as well. These allergies can even wind up causing episodes of rhinitis, conjunctivitis, and asthma attacks. Some people experience less serious irritation, but nevertheless find themselves undergoing treatment for part of the year.

What follows is some advice on curbing the presence of these intrusive creatures.

Keep an Eye on Your Bedding

Cleaning and efficiently ridding your house of dust is an excellent way to decrease the frequency of allergic episodes, but it isn't enough: give special consideration to bedding, starting with mattresses, which can house an impressive number of dust mites. A particularly effective means of protection from this kind of colonization is to thoroughly vacuum and hermetically seal your mattress in a specifically designed anti-dust mite plastic slipcase. The same goes for anti-dust mite pillow covers. Such products work by sealing in existing mites, starving them of their food: skin cells.

Dust mites, living and dead, together with their excrement, constitute an estimated 10 percent of the weight of your pillow. This figure alone should convince you to pay attention to your pillows. Does your pillow weigh two pounds? Then it may contain 3.5 ounces of dust mites. How can such an astonishing figure be explained? Bear in mind that humans shed, on average, 0.1 ounces of dead skin cells per night, or a little more than two pounds of squamae every year, not to mention quarts of sweat. Dust mites feed on skin cells and adore moisture, so your bedding provides choice lodgings for them. Regularly changing pillows is of obvious benefit, especially since pillows can also—in the days after a cold, for example—contain droplets of saliva.

To fight dust mites effectively, washing blankets, quilts, bedspreads, pillowcases, sheets, and bolsters every two weeks at temperatures of 160 degrees Fahrenheit or higher is recommended. Furthermore, people with allergies might opt for a bed frame with wooden or metal slats, since the fabric covering of box springs provides a good place for these tiny pests to make their homes.

Dust mites also nest in less-expected places, such as curtains, which should be cleaned at least once a year. Coats and clothes can also draw them, so these should be stored in closed containers. Upholstered furniture should be vacuumed with attention. Shoes can also play host to these allergen carriers and should not, in any case, be left in the bedroom.

A Bedroom Made for You, Not for Dust Mites

A bedroom is effectively a confined space where we spend at least a third of our time. The layout of your bedroom can be more or less favorable to the growth dust mites. Sticking to a few easy rules can help significantly reduce their presence while making your bedroom a healthier place on the whole.

In practical terms, avoid creating inaccessible corners or accumulating knickknacks that do nothing but collect dust. Why not take a page from Japanese interior design principles, which advocate keeping objects to a minimum? Going for smooth, unobstructed surfaces greatly facilitates cleaning, which should be performed with care by passing a moist cloth over furniture and objects daily. There's no point wearing yourself out cleaning if all it does is raise dust and get it moving around your room.

Vacuuming regularly is also important, but keep in mind that an ordinary vacuum multiplies the number of allergens in the surrounding air by a factor of five. Only a few models have proven themselves to be truly airtight: most spew out some of the very dust they've vacuumed in, which explains the multiplication of allergens. Fortunately, a solution exists: leave your windows open for one or two hours after vacuuming, and don't forget to change bags and filters regularly. If possible, use a machine with a HEPA filter.

To remain a healthy and comfortable environment, a bedroom must close its doors to certain guests: first of all, green plants, especially anywhere near the bed. Next, cats and dogs, as they are often carriers of dust mites. Allergies can, moreover, develop years after the introduction of a furred creature to the house.

Finally, it is important that the temperature of the room not be more than 68 degrees Fahrenheit, and that the humidity remain below 50 percent. Those susceptible to allergies should apply these same rules to every room of the house. There is no call, of course, to turn your home into an empty and impersonal space, but the rising number of dust-mite-related allergic episodes and severe asthma attacks gives cause for concern. Consequently, it is vital to rid your house of all unnecessarily dusty areas, which provide nesting grounds, and to give some thought to adjustments of habit and layout that will make daily cleaning easy and effective. Modern rules of hygiene necessitate devising sprucer habitats. You might call it a new lifestyle.

Germs Abroad

To travel is to die and be reborn every moment.
—VICTOR HUGO

In the last few years, travel has become much more accessible than before: organized tours with everything included now put the planet's most remote corners within easy reach. The marked increase in international air traffic, along with a decrease in fares, clearly illustrate this trend. But as travel has become widespread, so has disease. Germs have their native terrains: those prevalent in Asia and Africa often differ from those in Europe to such an extent that travelers expose themselves to dangers their bodies have never before encountered. This is of special concern in cases where no reliable vaccine exists.

Before leaping into a foreign adventure, it might be wise to take a few precautions.

Is There a Virus on Board?

Traveling is, above all, getting from place to place, which in itself poses health risks, not because of the possibility of accidents or motion sickness—against which rules of hygiene are quite ineffective—but because means of transport are confined spaces where many people are gathered. Such concentrations of people exponentially increase your chances of contracting diseases, especially aboard planes.

In the United States, John R. Balmes at the University of California has shown that 20 percent of people on long flights come down with colds in the five days that follow. Sometimes much more serious pathologies are passed on in the confined spaces of cabins. In 1996, a woman suffering from a resistant strain of tuberculosis flew from Chicago to Hawaii. Afterward, a third of the passengers seated in the two neighboring rows tested positive for TB. In 2003, twenty-two people contracted SARS (severe acute respiratory syndrome) on a flight from Hong Kong to Beijing. In only three hours, a single individual was able to infect passengers seated seven rows away.

Fortunately, these remain isolated cases, but they could certainly be made even rarer if masks were worn by people with diseases transmitted via the airways, so to speak—that is, by simply breathing. We in the West rarely use masks, which are very popular in Asia. Let us hope that, with recent awareness campaigns, our habits in the matter will evolve.

No Touristic Immunity

Upon arriving at his or her destination—with or without a cold—the traveler is exposed to another set of risks, largely through lack of familiarity with local infectious threats. While local populations display an immunity to microbes common on the scene, travelers lack this protection. The most famous example is the infamous "turista," which strikes newly arrived vacationers. In most cases, the victims have eaten the same food as the natives, who show no sign of intestinal unrest. The explanation for their discomfort is simple: travelers' digestive systems are ill-adapted to the organisms in local food that cause diarrhea and abdominal pain. These episodes, while not usually serious, can quickly ruin a vacation and, in extreme cases, turn life threatening.

To protect yourself, exercise caution about what goes into your mouth, be it food or drink. Think twice before drinking local water: ideally, you should drink only spring or mineral water from bottles opened before your eyes. When this is impossible, boiling the water or using purification tablets helps limit risks. When it comes to food, choose cooked over raw, even with fruits and vegetables, and definitely with meat and fish.

Up-to-Date Vaccinations

Every part of the world has its own health risks necessitating specific precautions, especially where vaccines are concerned. Bear in mind that diseases no longer common in our climate still thrive elsewhere. Vaccinations are therefore a must to prevent vacations from becoming nightmares. However, effective vaccines do not exist for all diseases.

The easiest way to stay informed of health risks is to consult your doctor or a travel clinic. These clinics, regularly kept abreast of infectious situations abroad, will be able to suggest the vaccines best suited to your destination. Be careful, however, not to put off your visit until the last minute, as some vaccines require an incubation period before becoming effective.

One example is the yellow fever vaccination, essential to visiting equatorial Africa and South America. The injection must take place at least ten days before departure in order to allow the immune system time to respond properly.

Other shots often advised for travelers include:

- hepatitis B (Africa and the Far East)
- hepatitis A (subtropical and tropical zones)
- BCG vaccine, against tuberculosis, tubercular meningitis, and miliary disease (all areas)
- meningitis and meningococcus (sub-Saharan Africa)
- Japanese encephalitis (Southeast Asia and rural India)
- typhoid (Southeast Asia, rural parts of Africa, the Caribbean, and South America)

Beware of Bilharziasis

You've probably never heard of bilharziasis (also called schistosomiasis), yet according to the World Health Organization, today this illness affects more than 200 million people. It is caused by a flatworm that lives inside a mud or freshwater snail. To avoid this flatworm, it's important not to swim just anywhere. Opt for treated pools or the open sea instead of rivers and standing water in lakes and ponds. Also beware of walking on mud or wet earth. These activities provide opportunities for the microscopic worm to attach itself to the skin with its sucker and then penetrate the body. Ten minutes are enough for it to reach a small blood vessel, and in four days it can reach the lungs. The bladder is often affected, which leads to frequent blood in the urine. Bilharziasis is rampant in many parts of the world, but mainly in Africa, in the Nile Valley, and in India, where a few pockets remain. Vigilance is essential in these regions.

Are You Up-to-Date?

Love is the vaccine for pride.
                              —FRIEDRICH HEBBEL

The invention of vaccination was a crucial step in the evolution of medicine. It allowed us to curb the spread of serious diseases such as rabies, polio, diphtheria, and tetanus. Yet it is important to remember that vaccines have a few disadvantages. First of all, they are quite difficult to develop. Faced with AIDS or avian flu, people naturally worry, the powers that be are moved to act, and charitable foundations do all they can to assemble the necessary funds for research. Everyone awaits the announcement of a vaccine that will at last solve the problem, but working out its exact composition can prove exceedingly difficult, requiring many years of study. In addition, in the case of emergent viruses such as the avian flu, we must wait for the first human-to-human transmission to occur before we can adapt a vaccine to humans, which will take at least six months. In the case of AIDS, after many, many years of research, and despite great advances, we still have a long way to go toward the development of a reliable formula.

Vaccines are at the heart of a paradox: once perfected and put on the market, they are used by only a small number of people. Some refuse them out of fear of side effects, others fail to get them out of simple negligence, and still others refuse them because they believe the disease in question will disappear from the planet, making vaccination pointless. The percentage of a given population vaccinated against an illness varies greatly from disease to disease and country to country for lack of a universal and obligatory vaccination standard.

We are quite right to wonder if we aren't in danger of seeing certain "eradicated" diseases reappear as epidemics. What are the facts, and where do the real risks lie? To gain a better understanding, let's look into smallpox.

Smallpox: A Question of Risk Management

Over the centuries, smallpox has taken a terrible toll worldwide. Because transmission is airborne, this disease proves quite contagious, like the flu, and deadly in a high number of instances. Some strains have a 90 percent mortality rate! A worldwide terrorist attack using smallpox could result in 2 to 3 million deaths. Other varieties are considered less dangerous but have severe aftereffects, especially where facial scarring is concerned.

However, smallpox vaccination, itself by no means

harmless, has lapsed on a global scale. Thanks to systematic injections, smallpox has almost completely vanished from the planet. Because the vaccine entails risks of side effects, and chances of an epidemic are now quite low, the reasons for this lapse are quite clear. But even so, there's no guarantee that the disease has disappeared. Smallpox may reemerge at any time and cause terrible damage.

Smallpox provides an interesting model with which to understand other vaccines. It all boils down to a question of the relationship between cost and effectiveness—in other words, the relationship between the possible side effects and the degree of protection a vaccine affords us, which depend on the disease's frequency and seriousness. Such a relationship is not always easy to quantify precisely, and brings into play parameters that are outside the scope of this discussion. Practically speaking, the easiest thing for both adults and children is to follow the recommendations of health authorities where vaccinations are concerned, and heed the established schedule of booster shots.

Self-Immunization

You can also immunize yourself against certain illnesses without specific vaccines. The most common and significant disease for which this can be done is toxoplasmosis. This illness is very dangerous in pregnant women, capable of causing birth defects. No vaccine exists, but if the mother-to-be has been exposed to the organism already during childhood or adolescence, from being in contact with cats, or from consuming undercooked meat on a regular basis, it is possible that she is naturally immune. A simple lab test will tell. If the results are negative, the pregnant woman should avoid keeping company with cats and abstain from raw or undercooked meat.

While this kind of natural immunization may help, good hygiene also includes being up-to-date on vaccinations that many adults tend to neglect. If you are among those guilty of letting your vaccinations slide, a quick look at your immunization booklet with your doctor can only do you good. You've been warned!

PART II

BON APPÉTIT!

As we have seen, travel, tourism, increasingly resistant germs and microbes, and a neglect of basic hygiene have given rise to new afflictions and allowed the resurgence of old ones. In the following section—unlikely to whet your appetite—we shall see that our work has been cut out for us and that, more and more, danger lurks in the dishes set before us.

Defending Your Life—with a Knife!

Bread has no say against the knife.
                    —GUADALOUPEAN PROVERB

A few years ago, while vacationing in Turkey, I had the chance to tour a fig farm. The sun was blazing and I was blinded by the glare on the white facades of the houses. The contrast was therefore all the more shocking when, pushing open the door to the room where the fruits were being prepared, I was plunged abruptly into darkness.

Nothing came to me from out of the shadows but, here and there, a little titter. Gradually my eyes began to make out shapes. I noted that my shirt had a violet tinge to it now: the room was flooded in blacklight, like a discotheque. Once I'd grown accustomed to this strange atmosphere, I made out a dozen or so young women, armed with knives, who seemed to be fiddling with figs. Drawing closer to them, I realized the reason for the lighting: the fluorescence brought out glowing patches on the skins of certain fruits. These carcinogenic patches, difficult to see with the unaided eye, are called aflatoxins.

"These parts are removed with knives since growers call for selective sorting to avoid lawsuits," explained Professor Jacques Estienne of the Center of Research and Development of Consumer Products in Marseille, France.

This example demonstrates that alimentary dangers are everywhere, even where we least expect them. Against some of these, a mere knife can be our best defense. We shall see how and why.

Organic Doesn't Mean Risk Free

Organic foods are a fine idea, founded on a more wholesome relationship with the earth and nature. However, its obligation is to the means, and not the results. Let me explain: to farm organically is to respect certain very specific guidelines that forbid, for instance, the use of certain chemical fertilizers. The label "organic" thus refers to production methods, not to the quality of the product obtained. If a farmer grows organic turnips at the bottom of a valley in a field exposed, from seepage, to chemical products from surrounding nonorganic fields above, his turnips are permitted to maintain their organic certification. The consumer suspects nothing.

Organic certification is not consistent internationally. As a result, we find for sale products marked "organic" whose chemical substance content can vary wildly. What's more, contrary to popular wisdom, there is no difference at a nutritional level between "organic" and other products: the levels of vitamins and other nutrients are the same.

To sum up, eating organic foods is a very worthy step to take, but is one more of philosophy than of nutrition or health. It can even turn problematic if the consumer, filled with confidence by the organic label, neglects the precautions basic to eating any fruit or vegetable. Take, for instance, an organically farmed apple. Apples are among the most well-liked organic produce. The problem is that molds like them too. Molds show up as brown spots on the skin of the fruit. Some of them secrete a dangerous toxin called patulin, a well-known carcinogen. All apples are exposed to such risks, but in conventional agriculture, the use of pesticides—in this case, fungicides—protects the fruit and curbs the growth of molds. Yet, for all that, it would be a pity to turn our backs on organically farmed apples. A very simple solution exists: before sinking your teeth into a crisp apple, organic or not, all you need to do is take a knife and remove the harmful brown spots.

Peel Your Fruits

The powers that be rightly remind us that fruits are very good for our health. How true—but their benefits derive from their high vitamin and fiber content rather than chemical additives. As we've seen with apples, the spraying of "contact" pesticides helps fight against all kinds of molds and insects. The downside is that these substances are often found on the skins of fruits. Ingesting them is a distinctly unhealthy act.

The average apple receives up to twenty successive chemical treatments. All you have to do to avoid them is peel the fruit before eating it, bearing in mind this important fact: Most of a fruit's vitamin content is found near its outer edge. Peel carefully and sparingly: that way, you'll benefit from the vitamins without suffering any detrimental effects from pesticides. Peeling a fruit reduces the pesticide residue by a factor of ten.

There are other reasons why peeling is necessary. Various studies conducted in the American Midwest brought to light a high incidence of certain types of cancer (notably brain, kidney, and pancreatic) among farmers using certain chemical products. In other words, the deleterious effects of pesticides are quite real, even if specific toxicity thresholds have yet to be precisely determined.

Careful washing and peeling of apples, pears, tomatoes, cucumbers, and other foods before eating may not always be enough, however. The "systemic" category of chemical product enters by absorption and travels throughout a plant's vascular stream. It can therefore be found in the nectar and flesh of fruits and vegetables. This is where an awareness of the conditions under which your food is produced becomes especially important.

Your Life, up in Smoke

Besides being a good time among friends, barbecues offer the advantage of cooking foods in a very healthy way, as fat melts away in the flames, leaving leaner meat. Healthy, that is, on one condition, however: that the the meat is not allowed to char. As with the cake bottoms and pizza edges, overcooked, blackened meats and fish are extremely carcinogenic. The blackened parts contain polycyclic aromatic hydrocarbides with a high tar content. Eating just a little one-inch piece of burned crust is the same as smoking no fewer than ten packs of cigarettes in terms of the amount of tar absorbed. In other words, better drop that habit of nibbling the burned parts on the pretext of cleaning your plate, as you're risking your health.

Use your knife to scrape off black parts and throw them away. If there are too many, it's better to eat something else, as the stakes are too high to be worth it. Ideally, you want to avoid the chemical "cracking" of the fatty hydrocarbons (which shows up as black points or lines) during cooking. A simple way to do this: invest in a quality grill and cook only over glowing embers of purified wood charcoal.

Also avoid grilling your racks of rib and shish kebabs right after adding fresh charcoal to hot embers: that's just asking for benzopyrene fumigation. Smoke flavor indeed!

The Benefits of Citrus

Asking for an orange from an apple tree is a common disorder.

—GUSTAVE FLAUBERT

C itrus fruits are rich in vitamins, fantastic for your health, and make delicious fresh juice. However, oranges, grapefruit, and lemons get their fair share of pesticides. How to keep the best and throw out the rest?

A Sensitive Subject

Where toxicology is concerned, everyone is different—meaning that, faced with the same danger, each organism reacts according to his or her genetic makeup. Genetic tests have highlighted gross inequalities, notably with regard to cancer: a gene for a predisposition to colon cancer (GSTM-1) has, for example, been discovered. People with this gene should avoid eating meat, since consumption of animal protein increases the risk of cancer. However, as only a small percentage of the population has this gene, it would be absurd for everyone to give up eating meat for this reason.

Another example is the hemoprotein cytochrome P450, which multiplies the risk of lung cancer in smokers by a factor of thirty. Here again, the number of people concerned is quite small. Variations in sensitivity like these demonstrate the need for treatments that are more focused or even individually tailored, so that people may enjoy lifestyles in accordance with their genetic makeup, and knowledge may be gained about the risks various lifestyles entail.

At the hour of this writing, scientists are far from having identified all the "at-risk" genes, and genetic testing is only conducted in very specific cases. Therefore, some of us who are particularly sensitive to the chemicals used in pesticides remain unaware of our vulnerability. One can avoid unnecessary risks by juicing oranges by hand, buying only citrus fruit that hasn't been chemically treated after harvesting, and foregoing that twist of lemon or lime garnish. In these ways, we can limit our daily exposure to toxins.

Put Those Electric Juicers Away

The pressure exerted by an electric juicer on the skin of an orange pushes pesticides from the periphery toward the heart of the fruit. As a result, chemicals may make their way into the juice. Better to rinse the fruit first, then get a bit of exercise juicing your fruits by hand. Squeeze them on a manual juice press—an act that, if practiced daily, will promote the development of wrist muscles. Freshly pressed fruit juice should be immediately consumed, in order to maximize the benefit of its vitamin C content, as vitamin C oxidizes quickly once exposed to light and air.

Mind the Rind!

Should you be served tea, soda, or another drink with a bit of decorative lemon peel dangling from the edge of the glass, remove it immediately, just as you would ice cubes in foreign countries, for peels, rinds, and zest present toxicological or microbial dangers. Harmful chemicals can easily make their way into a drink from a twist of lemon zest, and you would gulp them down being none the wiser. Pesticides are, as usual, at fault here. Lemons are treated with numerous products, including thiabendazole and benomyl, and ingesting these chemicals is far from advisable, as they may interfere with the functioning of the body's hormonal systems. While the dose from a single serving would be quite small, regular consumption magnifies the toxicity, just as with tobacco. We know that tobacco's impact on health depends a great deal more on how long-standing the habit is than on the quantity consumed daily. When you double your daily tobacco intake, you double your risk of cancer, whereas the same risk is magnified by twenty when the length of the habit of consumption is doubled. Just imagine what we may find out in twenty years about lemon peels!

Revenge of the Garçon

A man always has a right to revenge, no matter how small.

—GRAHAM GREENE

Mastering hygiene at home is essential, but it isn't always easy to do in the outside world, with groups, or in public places. Restaurants, for example, can be the source of many surprises. When a chef with a cold coughs on your *salade niçoise*, you can get a throat infection two days later.

Spitting: A Filthy Habit

Let's take a moment to examine the risks we run when, without our knowing it, a restaurant employee coughs over a platter or, worse, decides to take out their hostility for whatever reason by spitting on our food.

The danger depends on several parameters, starting with the time elapsed between the spraying of contaminated saliva on the platter and the moment when the platter is actually served. If only a few minutes go by, as in a table-service restaurant for example, the risk is much lower than it would be after two or three hours (a more common occurrence in cafeterias, buffets, and catered events). Microbial growth increases with the passing of time, until it attains what is known as the MID, or minimum infectious dose—that is, the number of germs needed to cause disease.

The kind of food is also important. Germs proliferate slowly in dry foods, but foods like mayonnaise and raw meats allow them to multiply more rapidly. Outside temperature is just as important: cold slows germ growth, while room temperature promotes it.

The revenge of the waiter (garçon) is for naught if he carries no disease. In the end, the danger depends on what state of health the person doing the spitting or coughing is in: if it's good, without signs of infection, there's no risk at all. If, on the other hand, that person has a viral condition such as a throat infection, there is a very real danger of passing it on.

Chefs or waiters who cough over your plate are but one example among many. Although many viruses do not last long outside the body, they can be found on a poorly washed glass, placemat, countertop, or teacup.

The Barbarous Tartare

Most smiling, smooth, detested parasites,
Courteous destroyers, affable wolves, meek bears,
You fools of fortune, trencher-friends, time's flies.
—WILLIAM SHAKESPEARE

Take a moment to picture an appetizing platter of carpaccio, rich and well-seasoned, beside a green salad. Tempting, isn't it? The catch is that in sampling it, you might just ingest a tapeworm larva. It looks like a tiny white dot, difficult to spot with the naked eye—you'd probably need a microscope above your plate—but then see it you would, with the four rounded suckers on its head that it uses to attach itself to your intestinal wall. You wouldn't notice anything upon swallowing it. No symptoms would present themselves until a few weeks later, by which time it would have grown into a ravenous white worm several yards long.

We've already examined, in an earlier chapter, some common intestinal parasites. Now let's take a closer look at what may be the most feared and famous of them all.

The Beef Tapeworm

The bovine tapeworm, *Taenia saginata*, is hermaphroditic—that is, it possesses a complete set of male and female reproductive organs. It can range in length from six to seventy-five feet as it grows inside the intestines. The common appellation "solitary tapeworm" is in fact a misnomer; it is not rare to find several tapeworms in the same intestine. Their lifespan is fairly long: they can live up to fifteen years in the absence of treatment.

Effective medications exist. From the number of treatments sold annually by French pharmaceutical manufacturers, the number of reported French cases can be extrapolated—between sixty thousand and one hundred thousand—but the number of actual cases may be even larger, since a sort of curtain of silence shrouds information on this condition. For some reason, tapeworms are widely regarded as shameful, and many people suffer in silence till the day they decide to consult a doctor for treatment. The problem can then be solved in a matter of weeks.

It is high time this silence was broken, since the symptoms of tapeworm infection are numerous and daily troublesome, first of all because the worm sheds small segments, about the size of a grain of rice, signaling its presence. The average tapeworm possesses more than a thousand such segments and can shed four to twenty per day, each containing fifty thousand to eighty thousand eggs! Finding the segments in one's stool is never a pleasant experience, and the other symptoms are even less so: fatigue, digestive problems, bloating, nausea, fullness and loss of appetite, and diarrhea.

In some cases, patients complain of persistent anal itching and a constant agitated state. Asthma attacks have even been triggered by the presence of this parasite. These diverse symptoms are sometimes wrongly attributed to emotional instability or psychological problems. So long as the condition has not been clearly diagnosed, the patient is forced to suffer these inconveniences in silence. Only by fully detailing such symptoms to their doctors can patients expect them to be properly addressed.

The only advantage to the tapeworm—if it can be termed an advantage—is that it causes weight loss, sometimes up to twenty-two pounds. Urban legend has it that an unscrupulous company packaged the little white worms in glass capsules and marketed them as weight-loss products. Indeed, after swallowing the worms, people would lose weight—but what a price to pay! The diet scene is regularly flooded with dangerous gimmicks. Whether amphetamines, diuretics, or thyroid extracts, over the past twenty years many weight-loss products have exposed users to major health risks. The sale of tapeworms seems like only one of many profoundly unprincipled practices.

Tapeworms are parasites to be gotten rid of without delay, even if it means keeping a couple of extra pounds. Diagnosis is not always easy, given the shameful silence often associated with the disease, and the fact that the egg-bearing segments are not always easy to spot. Doctors can use a cellophane-tape swab to examine the perineal area. Segments will stick to the cellophane, allowing doctors to confirm the parasite's presence.

Treatment then consists of an anthelmintic or vermicide, designed to kill the worm so that it may be flushed from the system. Be aware, however, that most such drugs are contraindicated in several instances, especially for pregnant women. Mothers-to-be, and the rest of us, would do well to keep in mind the importance of preventive hygiene.

How Tapeworms Can Be Avoided

One simple, basic rule is that beef should be frozen for at least ten days before being consumed raw. Just to be safe, it is advisable to also freeze beef that will eventually be cooked, since only steak cooked medium or well done (140 degrees Fahrenheit) ensures the elimination of tapeworms. The problem is that many people prefer their steak rare or medium rare. Searing a nice thick filet mignon on the outside but leaving it bloody within in no way reduces the risk of contracting a tapeworm. Given that many Americans are beginning to try carpaccio, and remain partial to their steak, tapeworms pose a real threat.

Marinating beef in brine is not very effective: only a solution of at least 20 percent salt for more than five days will succeed in killing off tapeworms. Although consumers worry over ionizing radiation, they are wrong to do so: It is effective in getting rid of tapeworms and other food-borne pathogens.

The surest way to eliminate tapeworms in beef at home is to freeze it before eating: The worm cannot survive temperatures of 13 degrees Fahrenheit or lower for more than ten days. This simple practice permits us to enjoy beef in all its forms, from raw to well done. Be careful: Simply chilling a cut of beef in order to slice it more easily into carpaccio is not enough. Only prolonged freezing is effective.

Teaching a Man to Eat Fish

> I'm a Pisces with a mayonnaise ascendant.
> —ETTORE SCOLA

One morning in January 2006, a young Icelander woke up with an intense itching sensation in his throat. Although he coughed harder and harder, the sensation persisted. He ended up, with the help of a lamp and a mirror, looking into his mouth, where he discovered, to his horror, a white worm two inches in length squirming at the back of it. Six days earlier, he had unknowingly swallowed a parasite, *Anisakis,* while eating inadequately cooked fish. Terrifying, isn't it? Indeed, yet in fact also quite common. In this case, the young man was lucky enough to have the parasite removed before it could cause damage to his digestive tract.

Others have been less fortunate. A few months later, an Italian was admitted to the ER for appendicitis. Surgery revealed a perforated cecal wall—part of the large intestine—the dead tissue was removed and a resection of the necrotized area was performed. What caused the perforation? Raw anchovies, believed to be carriers of the *Anisakis* worm, consumed several days earlier.

A Formidable Intestinal Foe

Humans become infected with *Anisakis* worms by ingesting larva in raw fish. The parasites then make themselves at home in the stomach or intestine. Fish affected are, among others, herring, sardines, and mackerels from the English Channel, the North Sea, the Atlantic Ocean, and the waters of the Far East. *Anisakis* is found in fish from the wild but rarely in farmed fish. For once, cheaper is also safer.

Every year, groups of raw-fish lovers find themselves in emergency surgery because of this little parasite. *Anisakis* causes anisakiasis, a disease leading to intestinal perforations that can trigger many potentially deadly complications, such as peritonitis and septicemia. Yet anisakiasis is often difficult to diagnose, since it is not the first thing to occur to doctors. Victims generally complain of sometimes violent abdominal pain, nausea, and bowel difficulties, symptoms, similar to those of other intestinal disorders.

Several factors, however, point to the worm as the cause, one of them being elevated eosinophil counts in blood samples. Eosinophils are a type of white blood cell whose increased count betrays the presence of a parasite or an allergic reaction. A gastrointestinal endoscopy and a biopsy under general anesthesia also allow doctors to determine the presence of anisakis.

Sometimes intestinal perforations are discovered only at the stage of emergency surgical intervention, often during an exploratory laparotomy—that is, an operation opening the abdomen to examine it. This has been noted by M. J. Ramos and his research teams at the General Hospital of LaVega Baja in Spain, where it became routine to ask patients who presented symptoms requiring gastrointestinal surgery whether they had eaten raw fish in the preceding weeks.

Conventional anthelmintic treatments (worm medicines) are not effective against anisakis. Surgeons use endoscopy and extract the parasite with surgical pliers.

Faced with a dangerous parasite that is difficult to spot and treat, prevention is naturally the best remedy. Certain sanitary procedures must be followed from the time fish are caught. Fish must be immediately gutted and quickly frozen, forty-eight hours of freezing sufficing to destroy anisakis. Cooking the fish thoroughly is also effective, but it would be a pity to quash the current craze for raw fish—a fine idea since, generally speaking, the rawer a foodstuff, the greater its nutritional content: vitamins and fatty acids are often damaged by cooking.

Fish should be systematically frozen prior to consumption. From a regulatory point of view, this is inevitable: sushi must be prepared from frozen fish. At home, this is easy to ensure, but when eating out, one must visit a trusted restaurateur, or resort to sushi made with cooked fish. However, these rules are little respected, as certain experts believe that frozen fish loses much of its flavor.

Ciguatera

Fish can contain, in addition to parasites like anisakis, toxins such as ciguatera. Ciguatera poisoning is quite common, especially in tropical areas such as the Caribbean, Hawaii, Florida, and more generally the Indian and Pacific Oceans. It comes from a microalga (the dinoflagellate *Gambierdiscus toxicus*) that is dangerous to humans but is part of the diet of reef fish. These reef fish are consumed by larger predators, which are themselves consumed by human beings. The problem is that the toxin is resistant to high temperatures—that is, it is unaffected by cooking.

Symptoms can appear anywhere from a few minutes to a day and a half after ingestion, and include not only diarrhea, vomiting, dizziness, and paralysis, but also a markedly less common phenomenon: cold allodynia, or a burning sensation upon contact with cold. In addition, blood pressure drops and the pulse slows. Complications are occasionally life threatening, notably in the case of respiratory muscle paralysis. One to two cases out of every hundred end in death.

In order to avoid ingesting ciguatera, follow precautions when consuming fish by the seaside. Among suspect fish are carnivorous species of great age and size, such as barracuda, grouper, and reef dwellers such as parrotfish. Avoid consuming the heads and organs of these species. I recommend investigating the habits of natives—who, from experience, never eat certain kinds of fish—and following suit.

Watch Out for Histamine

Some fish, even without toxins and anisakis, are dangerous when they begin to spoil. They release histamine, a substance that, in small doses, is involved in the functioning of our immune systems. When absorbed in too high a quantity, it may cause serious allergic reactions. A high level of histamine in a fish betrays a lack of freshness, though this may not be noticeable in odor or taste.

Histamine comes from histidine, an amino acid particularly abundant in the blood of certain fish, especially red tuna. Tuna is thus the main culprit, but other fish such as rays and mackerel are just as dangerous. As with ciguatera, cooking does not get rid of histamine. Histamine poisoning is likely to lead to diarrhea and vomiting, skin flushing, itching, and palpitations. These signs, which appear immediately or up to three hours after ingestion, can last from several hours to several days.

Again, basic hygienic measures can prevent this kind of poisoning, starting with proper refrigeration. A few preventive practices have been implemented by fish farmers. These precautions appreciably decrease the risk involved, so long as fish are kept in the proper conditions before reaching your plate:

- Tuna are bled and gutted as quickly and cleanly as possible after capture, with a view to eliminating germs and blood, which contains histidine.
- Histamine levels are measured in large tuna before they are sold.
- Fish are kept on ice, which helps curb bacterial growth.

Suspect fish often has a characteristically peppery taste. At the slightest suspicion—whether from the fish's smell, look, or taste—be prudent and refrain from eating it.

Heavy Metals: Myth or Fact?

Heavy-metal toxicity in fish has been the subject of many debates, and it isn't always easy to get a clear picture of the facts. On one hand, regular consumption of fish is recommended—and rightly so, given the benefits of omega-3 fatty acids; on the other, there is the risk of absorbing high amounts of mercury and other toxic heavy metals. In truth, the goal should be, above all, to maintain balance and diversity.

It is true that predatory fish are virtual indexes of pollutants, especially mercury. Some have the capacity to concentrate mercury contained in the water, while others such as tuna, pike, and swordfish in particular are prone to accumulations of this pollutant because of their fattiness and large size. Being at the top of the marine food chain, tuna and swordfish have a high mercury content because they've eaten other, smaller, fish, which have in turn swallowed zooplankton, which themselves feed on contaminated phytoplankton.

Another factor: the mercury present in fish is extremely toxic to humans because it is by nature organic (methylmercury and ethylmercury). Fish are the principal source of this toxic element for humans: 80 percent of the methylmercury that we take in comes from fish, 10 percent from water, and 10 percent from elsewhere. This is why authorities have seen fit to determine heavy-metal levels in fish species by species.

Pollutant levels vary greatly from one fish to another. Right now, the Canadian government advises, for example, to "limit consumption of swordfish, shark, and fresh and frozen tuna to one meal per week. Pregnant women, women of childbearing age and young children should eat no more than one such meal per month."

It is not a matter of banning fish from our diet, since that would deprive us of its many benefits, but rather of limiting the consumption of certain species. Regular tuna eaters are advised, for example, not to exceed seven ounces per week.

The solution lies in maintaining balance and diversity. In general, the best practice would be to vary the species consumed as much as possible, in order not only to limit exposure to a single pollutant, but also to profit from the specific nutritional benefits of each kind of fish.

Shellfish

Like predatory fish, shellfish are indexes of pollutants: lead, cadmium, mercury, and other toxic substances can often be found in their flesh. Mollusks act as filters, collecting the many pollutants present in seawater. Any temporary pollution in a given zone shows up immediately as an increase in toxicity levels among harvested shellfish. The concentrations of toxic substances vary depending on species and origin. Oysters, for instance, contain four times as much cadmium and half as much lead as mussels. Moreover, pollutant levels vary by season. In the summer, milky oysters at the height of their maturity are lower in cadmium than in the winter.

Scallops, too, contain their share of pollutants, especially the orange tongue or coral scallop. A digestive organ, the coral scallop concentrates heavy metals, so it is better to remove it before eating scallops. Scallops are usually sold and served with the corals already removed in the United States, but this is not the case in Europe.

Bear in mind that pollutants found in fish or shellfish

usually come from human beings. The best way for humankind to lessen the danger linked with fish and shellfish consumption is to cut down on the pollution of our oceans. It would be a great pity, for fear of toxic substances, to be forced to give up eating shellfish.

The Dangers of Salad

I am not a vegetarian because I love animals; I am a
vegetarian because I hate plants.

—A. Whitney Brown

Every year, the seemingly innocent activity of eating
lamb's lettuce (mâche) or watercress lands people in
hospital hepatology clinics, because they have contracted
from these terrifically healthy salad staples an illness running rampant in several countries. Called hepatic distom-
atosis or fasciolosis, it is better known by its carrier/host,
the common liver fluke.

The parasite, *Fasciola hepatica*, frequently infests sheep
but also cows and steers. What do these have to do with salads? Well, the parasite lives in the animal's bile ducts, regularly laying eggs that are then passed in dung. Once on
the ground, these eggs hatch in conditions of moisture,
continuing a parasitic cycle and freeing larva that attach
themselves to surrounding vegetation, paving the way for
possible human consumption. Humans can contract liver
flukes by eating "wild" salad greens picked near contami-

nated pastures. The vegetables most often to blame are lamb's lettuce, watercress, and dandelion greens.

The current "back-to-nature" trend drives many city dwellers to set off on a quest for healthier, more natural products said to be risk-free. Weekends in the country allow them to rediscover the joys of the harvest. The impression of being healthy by eating foods without pesticides, nitrates, chemical additives, or other industrial products can create a liberating sensation. However, not everything in nature is necessarily healthy. The intervention of chemical substances is sometimes preferable, as I explained in the case of apples (see the chapter titled "Defending Your Life—with a Knife!").

Where liver flukes are concerned, it's clear that picking your own salads in the wild can be quite dangerous, as this pathology is far from benign, and its symptoms do not always immediately manifest themselves. Sometimes up to three weeks may pass between consumption of the contaminated food and the appearance of the first signs: fevers accompanied by overall changes; abdominal pain, especially along the right side; and urticaria, or hives. All this is but a primary stage which, in some cases, doesn't even occur.

Three to six months later, things are different. The subject complains of liver pain and low-grade fever. Often he or she will appear jaundiced, the light yellow tint of this condition most easily observed in the eyes. At this stage, the parasite has set up shop in the liver and caused an infection of the bile ducts. Painful attacks of biliary colic follow.

It is possible to diagnose fasciolosis as early as the third week, through immunological blood tests. One stage later, the parasite's brown eggs can be found in the patient's stool. Treatment with triclabendazole, available in pharmacies, can help rid the patient's system of them. The earlier the drugs are prescribed, the more effective they will be. The treatment generally runs at least ten days and requires multiple precautions. Sometimes surgery will be necessary if faced with a liver abscess, jaundice of prolonged duration, or cholangitis, an inflammation of the bile ducts, resistant to prescribed dosages. Secondary cirrhosis of the liver is quite rare given advances in medication.

It is preferable by far to avoid contracting a liver fluke by leaving wild salad greens alone. When washing salads, clean the leaves individually instead of plunging them all into the same water. This will remove a maximum of undesirable elements while preserving nutrients.

New and Emerging
Vectors of Disease

One man's meat is another man's poison.
                                    —PARACELSUS

The rise in the virulence of food-borne illnesses may be traced to several sources. The globalization of the food supply is the first to spring to mind. In 1997, there was a North American outbreak of cyclospora, spread on a large scale by raspberries imported from South America. Subjects suffered from diarrhea, and parasites were found in their stool. Air transport and modern logistics had allowed fruit from all four corners of the world to reach our local supermarkets.

We put much more trust in food bought in our favorite neighborhood store than in a foreign country. A tourist in an unfamiliar country doubtless takes a thousand tiny precautions before eating so much as a piece of fruit, from fear of contracting disease, yet we don't question locally available produce. It just so happens the very same fruits are distributed to both European and American markets, and they are often teeming with parasites. To avoid nasty surprises, we should very carefully wash all fruits and vegetables, rinsing at least twice, or peel them before eating.

Examples of contamination are many. Shoppers are pleased to find berries in supermarkets year-round, for example, yet the price they pay can prove hard to swallow. In Michigan, 153 cases of hepatitis A were linked to inadequately washed strawberries from Mexico in 1997. In addition, fruits and vegetables can, once in a refrigerator, contaminate neighboring foods if they are not cleaned and put away properly in separate compartments or sealed containers.

Diverse Factors

Foods are not the only vectors of emerging diseases, whose origins are in fact numerous. Take, for example, the aforementioned vibrio that is responsible for cholera. In 1991, a massive freighter discharge of contaminated ballast water* dramatically spread the organism in the southern coastal waters of the United States. During an ecological disaster such as an oil slick, attention is focused on toxicological dangers, but microbiological damage is just as serious.

Another contributing factor to the global spread of diseases is today's significant population migration, which

---

*The South American cholera outbreak of the early 1990s may be traced to a similar incident.

results in an incredible "stir" of germs. Whether tourists or immigrants, groups of people changing habits and places cause new outbreaks to arise. For instance, a 2006 study conducted by the Swedish Institute for Infectious Disease Control found that 90 percent of Swedish cases of salmonella were "imported"—that is, brought back to Sweden by residents from abroad. The intestinal flora of a given country's inhabitants are not always adapted to the culinary customs of the culture they move to or visit. These disparities increase vulnerability to many germs and parasites. If you experience digestive trouble such as prolonged diarrhea upon returning from a trip, have your stool examined for undesirable guests.

Other factors must also be taken into account: malnutrition among certain populations, which leaves them weakened and more vulnerable to infection, and lifestyle issues such as having lunch on the go, gulping down meals sometimes prepared in unsanitary conditions.

A Brief Survey of the Most Common Emerging Food-Borne Diseases

A certain number of pathologies are considered emergent either because they are new, or because instances of alimentary transmission were hitherto unknown. Some have shown themselves particularly formidable, beginning with *Listeria monocytogenes*, which was recently listed as "emerging" after the discovery that it could be transmitted by food. Normally, cold halts germ growth, but this little infectious bacillus has a unique feature: it is capable of growing and multiplying even in a refrigerator, at temperatures low as 35.6 degrees Fahrenheit. Although its growth is slowed, it eventually reaches the MID (minimum infective dose). Thus a food initially contaminated with *Listeria* in insufficient quantities to cause any symptoms can, even if properly refrigerated, become harmful as time goes by. Ingesting the food can result in listeriosis after an incubation period of about a week. The disease manifests itself in flulike symptoms, sometimes with fever, though these can be mild and often go unnoticed in adults in good health. Serious complications can arise, such as meningitis or meningoencephalitis, which are likely to endanger the patient's life or have severe neurological repercussions.

In pregnant women, the disease will appear as a simple flulike fever or minor digestive trouble. Sometimes, mothers-to-be will show no symptoms at all, and the pathology will not be discovered until an early miscarriage occurs. Neonatal listeriosis is responsible for 7 percent of infections among newborns.

Treatment consists of antibiotics which, in order to be effective, must be prescribed early on, or at any rate before serious complications develop. This is why it is important to remain attentive to any broadcasts from the authorities about new or recent cases of listeriosis or urging the recall of culpable products from the shelves. Often, lacking specific information, the patient or doctor will not consider listeriosis when faced with a low-grade, flulike fever. Public announcement of a recent outbreak can help establish the link between the presence of this bacillus and the symptoms it causes, as well as encourage rapid antibiotic treatment. In such cases, not alerting the public or failing to instigate a recall of a contaminated product would be tantamount to not helping a person in danger. Unlike purchasers of, say, prescriptions or cars, purchasers of a given food item from a store cannot be tracked down. In the absence of a means of contacting individual consumers directly, we must rely on the media and individual vigilance to help check the spread of disease.

Trematodes (from the Greek *trema*, meaning "hole"), or flukes, are also classified as a cause of emerging disease. They are primarily found in Southeast Asia and South America, but as foods and tourists crisscross the world, these seemingly distant pathologies have entered our daily orbit. The Swiss Tropical Institute estimates that 40 million people in the world are affected by trematodes, the source of many acute liver conditions that can lead to cancer. The new wave of trematodes can be explained by the consumption of aquaculture-farmed products and inadequately cooked freshwater fish.

No overview would be complete without mentioning "mad cow" disease. BSE (bovine spongiform encephalopathy) was discovered in Great Britain in 1985, but not until 1995 was it suspected that this animal disease could be passed on to human beings. Scientists dubbed the human form "a new variation on Creutzfeldt-Jakob disease,"* and it caused a world health scare that everyone no doubt remembers, with a reported 120 people contracting this illness. Health authorities and the food industry have taken prevention as far as they can, but this pathology has not, for the moment, disappeared. This disease results in death, as there is as yet no effective treatment.

What Can We Do Against Emerging Diseases?

To fight all these recent pathologies and, as much as possible, contain their spread, serious preventive measures are called for at various levels.

First of all, thorough cooking of all meats and fish is recommended, especially ground meat, which is highly susceptible to microbial dangers. To understand why, all you have to do is spread out your ground meat. You will find that its exposed surface area, with all its involutions, is much greater than that of solid slabs or cuts. This should give you an idea of the increased chance for possible contact between ground meat and external contaminants: unlike a single cut of meat, which is compact and less permeable, ground meat is choice terrain for microbes. The muscle fibers that are cut during grinding further increase the risk. The solution? Consume ground meat as soon as possible after purchase

---

*This disease already existed, but its manifestations and causes were different. The link with beef has not yet been established.

and cook it thoroughly. As for fresh herbs and vegetables—whether as seasoning, side dish, or entrée—it is important to clean them well before consumption.

Next, the kitchen itself must be immaculate, beginning with an element too often neglected: the refrigerator. It is frankly incredible how rarely certain appliances get cleaned. Keeping your food in a dirty refrigerator is like keeping your food on dirty plates! Refrigerators should be wiped down every two weeks with bleach- or vinegar-and-water compound. Moreover, it is important to organize your refrigerator so that raw foods do not come into contact with cooked foods ready to be consumed.

Not letting leftovers age in the fridge is another good instinct when it comes to food safety.* Knowing when to throw something out is knowing how to protect yourself. The longer you keep food around, the more germs it grows; some products, like fresh mayonnaise, are tantamount to a petri dish. It is best to consume foods directly after cooking them and get rid of the leftovers.

Another essential habit: wash your hands thoroughly before cooking and after handling raw items. Wooden cutting boards should be avoided, as microbes will thrive in their numerous crevices even if the boards are washed after use.

The prevention of infection is also a question of ergonomics: infectious agents find accommodation in hard-to-clean

---

*Let me add that, contrary to received wisdom, the act of reheating leftovers in a microwave oven in no way constitutes sterilization.

places. Certain household appliance manufacturers have finally begun to take this into consideration, giving preference to smooth curves instead of inaccessible corners, coming up with products that are easily cleaned or disassembled.

Don't forget that dish towels must be changed regularly. A wet, soiled towel cleans nothing—indeed, it is an ideal breeding ground for bacteria! Using such a towel simply recontaminates the object, food, or surface just cleaned instead of drying it. To avoid this, use disposable paper towels—certainly the most hygienic replacement for their fabric counterparts.

What to say about sponges? The average kitchen sponge houses 7.2 billion bacteria. An astronomical figure, which should lead to a simple habit: clean your sponges after use and replace them as often as possible.

Your trash can should be cleaned carefully at least once a week with bleach, lest it become a source of bacterial contamination in relative proximity to food.

Let me end this chapter by reminding readers of a few foods pregnant women should avoid: soft raw-milk cheeses, smoked fish, raw sprouted seeds, raw shellfish, and European charcuterie, especially potted meats. Other healthy individuals may consume these foods without danger, so long as they do so hygienically.

Salmonella and *Escherichia coli*

Man, too, is a stubborn microbe.

—JEAN GIONO

T here are many other food-borne diseases besides those already listed in this work. Most are well-known and health authorities have, with the help of the food-processing industry, been able to put in place measures that reduce the number of cases. Two parasites stand out from the rest: salmonella and the bacterium *Escherichia coli* serotype 0157:H7.

Humans and Salmonella: A Long History

Salmonella is a genus, all the members of which are gram-negative enterobacteria (meaning they don't hold Gram's purple dye when stained). These widespread germs cause salmonellosis, an illness always at the top of the food-poisoning charts, representing no less than 50 percent of reported cases! This figure is indeed worrisome, especially for young children and the elderly, to whom these parasites have proved life-threatening.

There have long been pockets of salmonella subsisting not only in animals (birds, ruminants, swine, rodents), but also in humans, among whom can be found "asymptomatic" carriers, who can pass the germs on to those around them. People who suffer from immunity deficiencies are at especially high risk. In addition, recent studies have found subjects with a genetic susceptibility to salmonella.

Contamination generally occurs via such foods as poorly preserved or undercooked eggs, ground meat, or chicken. Foodstuffs may contain a few salmonella without making people sick: As with any disease, the minimum infectious dose (MID) must be reached—in this case, around 100,000 bacteria per gram. Bear in mind that foods kept at room temperature have every chance of reaching this infectious dose.

The first symptoms of infection, which include diarrhea, vomiting, and fever, appear anywhere from six hours to three days after ingestion. Complications are rare—meningitis, brain or spleen abscesses—but salmonella symptoms, especially severe dehydration, can be quite dangerous to young children and the elderly.

In group settings, the discovery of a significant number of cases with similar symptoms helps point toward a diagnosis, which can subsequently be confirmed by tests. Antibiotic treatments have shown themselves to be quite effective. Any cases of group infection, such as at a school or retirement home, should be reported to the authorities.

As no vaccine exists, the three golden rules of hygiene remain our best preventive defense: hand washing, proper refrigeration, and thorough cooking of foods. Ultimately, the fight against salmonella also requires testing foodstuffs at various points along the production line. The powers that be thus have their part to play in the battle. This is every bit as true for another, more serious, threat: E. coli.

E. coli 0157:H7: A Bacterial Agent Licensed to Kill

This pathogenic agent was discovered in 1919. It was already making waves then, but it wasn't until 1982 that the Centers for Disease Control and Prevention brought its food-borne transmission to light, ushering *Escherichia coli* 0157:H7 into the pantheon of the most dangerous food-borne diseases. This very virulent bacterial strain causes bloody diarrhea and acute kidney failure, which can be fatal to children, or lead to serious repercussions later in life. In 1996, more than six thousand Japanese schoolchildren were affected, and two died. From Africa to Australia, from Europe to the Americas, the entire world has reason to be concerned about this microbe.

The bacterium is often linked to hamburgers in America, as it was found in ground meat in 1982. Since then, the number of cases has multiplied, sometimes taking disquieting proportions, as in the fall of 2005, when sixty-nine people were taken ill in the southwestern United States after eating ground beef. According to an article in *Emerging*

Infectious Diseases, currently 15 percent of American children have already been infected by E. coli, causing 7,500 cases of serious complications yearly.

In addition, this bacteria has a feature that makes it especially dangerous: unlike salmonella, for example, the MID is quite low—just a few dozen bacteria suffice. After an average incubation period of four days, these few bacteria can produce relatively benign symptoms such as watery stool, or sometimes more serious conditions, such as hemorrhagic colitis or acute, life-threatening kidney failure. The mortality rate ranges from 2 to 7 percent.

Ignorance of or disregard for the rules of hygiene in part explains the return of this microbial agent which, every year, claims victims around the world. This germ was already around a century ago, but the food-processing industry as we know it was not. Today, a single contaminated lot of any given foodstuff may reach thousands of consumers. Industries have put safety measures in place that are meticulous but not infallible; consumers need to do their part to avoid the mistakes that give these bacteria a chance.

The number of cases of infection has been rising for about twenty years, and not only in North America. The guilty foodstuffs are many: ground beef, unpasteurized fruit juice or milk, poorly washed lettuce, raw vegetables, drinking water, game, among other items. Ground beef is still the number-one cause. Cooking destroys the bacteria if it is thorough. Some of the foods above—lettuce or fruit juice, for example—are normally not cooked.

These preventive measures can effectively limit the risk of infection:

- Cook meats thoroughly, especially ground beef.
- Wash vegetables, fruits, and especially herbs with care, as the last are less often thought of as vectors of disease.
- Separate raw foods from cooked in the refrigerator.
- Reheat leftovers sufficiently and don't keep them for more than two to three days.
- Throw out the remains of any foods that spoil easily.
- Clean and dry kitchen implements and counter-tops after each use.
- Always wash your hands thoroughly before preparing meals, after handling raw foods, and after using the bathroom.

Two other important rules must be added to these oft-repeated ones. First of all, people suffering from gastroenteritis should not use swimming pools or public baths, and should in no case be allowed to cook for others. Next, I recommend keeping children under the age of five from contact with cows, calves, sheep, and goats, from which they run the risk of catching potentially dangerous germs.

PART III

PANIC ROOMS

"I knew a time when the main source of pollution was from people beating their rugs out the window," wrote Gilbert Cesbron. Today, pollutants are everywhere, and protecting the environment is a major concern on a global scale. But the dangers to our health in our very own hearths and homes cannot be overlooked. Just like the food on our plates, the rooms we live in can contain a host of pathogenic agents. These are more diverse and numerous than before; to combat them we must adapt our habits and adopt new rules of hygiene.

Hygiene at the Hospital

The hospital is a public establishment where sick people get to have their say.

—SERGE MIRJEAN

Nosocomial infections are ailments acquired by a patient from the very place where he or she goes to get treated for something else. They are generally caused by microorganisms (bacteria, viruses, or fungi) and affect all health institutions.

Understanding and Combating Nosocomial Infections

The idea that the hospital, whose purpose is to cure or to provide care, can also cause illness seems at first counterintuitive if not incomprehensible. Yet a hospital today with a 0 percent nosocomial infection rate is just as inconceivable. Such an institution would have to admit only patients in good health who came complaining of momentary fatigue, temporary asthenia, fleeting anorexia, or sporadic bouts of melancholy—and not even then would the risk be completely absent!

Three basic facts are crucial to a full understanding of this phenomenon. First, take a look at the makeup of the hospitalized population, which includes a significant number of the elderly. As a group, they are regularly hospitalized. As mentioned in an earlier chapter, the immune system gets less and less effective with age, and susceptibility to infections increases, just as it does for the HIV-positive, those receiving long-course chemotherapy, and diabetics.

Second, common sense tells us that many patients come to the hospital precisely because they are already suffering from highly contagious infectious diseases.

Third, a health institution is a closed environment.

These three facts—a susceptible population, a significant concentration of pathogenic agents, and a closed environment—are largely responsible for the propagation of nosocomial infections. Add to these that medicine is progressing by leaps and bounds, necessitating a constant redefinition of what constitute sanitary measures and hygienic practices. Doctors must treat ever more fragile patients with ever more complex techniques. Highlighting the pace of innovation and its demands serves to emphasize an extremely important point: sometimes, no one is at fault. Nosocomial infections can result from phenomena as yet unknown to doctors. Advances in medicine continue to increase life expectancy. The elderly will continue to be more susceptible to infection than younger people, while new viruses will appear for which no treatment or vaccine yet exists. The medical profession will be forced to discover new remedies.

What truly matters here is to take into account nosocomial infections that can be prevented. Some of them result from a failure to follow proper sanitary procedures, which is unacceptable: for example, bacteria from a building's water supply contaminating a surgical unit, or the transmission of a virus via endoscopic or surgical tools. It is important to maintain, even intensify, efforts to avoid this kind of accident, all the more so as nosocomial infections offer a model, in miniature, of what lies in store.

Everyone Up!

The issues associated with bed rest are well known in hospitals. The longer a patient stays in bed, the higher the risk of mortality, simply from not walking around. Venous stasis provokes phlebitis (inflammation of the veins), which in turn can cause pulmonary embolisms (arterial blockage in the lungs). In order to prevent such complications, anticoagulants (blood thinners) are usually administered while a patient is bedridden, and the hospital stay is frequently reduced. Thus, while pregnant women might have once remained in the hospital for up to ten days, today they are out in three or fewer if no complications arise. Older medical manuals describe a problem observed on the eighth day, when the young mother attempts to rise from bed: "After one week of bed rest, she rises, pales, gives out a cry, and falls to the floor." The cause? A massive, possibly deadly pulmonary embolism due to prolonged bed rest.

Assisted Living

As people age, their autonomy tends to decrease, until the day when their families—often starting with their own children—raise the idea, with the best of intentions, that they should perhaps no longer live alone.

People living on their own sometimes run fewer risks than those living in a group. The immune system decreases in efficacy with age, putting the elderly as a population at higher risk from infectious diseases. Therefore, when a hundred or so seniors are cut off from the outside world, a phenomenon common to day cares and elementary schools arises: Someone is always getting everyone else sick. Life in a high-density community promotes the transmission of contagious diseases, which can be dangerous to the elderly.

Moreover, prolonged inactivity is, in and of itself, a source of multiple complications. Thromboembolic accidents, such as phlebitis or pulmonary embolisms, are more common in inactive individuals; muscle mass wastes away more quickly and bones become brittle. No longer having to manage their lives or look out for themselves often sets the elderly down a slippery slope in which they let themselves go, faring less and less well against such relatively ordinary stresses as the common cold. If we took the time to compare statistically the very real danger of an elderly person alone at home falling and hurting themselves with the increased mortality rate of living in a closed environment like a retirement home, we would not hesitate to run the risk of letting the elderly live in their own homes whenever possible.

A Treasure Trove of Effective Measures

On the subject of nosocomial infections, much remains to be said that lies perhaps beyond the scope of this book; yet the struggle against such infections is among this book's core themes. We will see that the basic preventive measures against these kinds of infections are adapatable or transposable to our own lives.

Note that in certain sensitive hospital environments, visitors are required to slip paper covers on their shoes. The point of this is simple: to keep outside germs from making their way in. In the outside world, streets and sidewalks are veritable jungles of germs, with litter but one of the particularly virulent flora to be found there, not to mention the excrement of dogs and birds.

Of course, no one would be so crazy as to lick the sidewalk, nor would they eat a morsel of food dropped in the street, but imagine, for a moment, that a particularly harmful microbe manages to infiltrate an apartment on the sole of a shoe. If it has rained, dampness creates a milieu favorable to the development of viruses on the ground. Now suppose that a child drops a toy on the floor, it gets contaminated, and the child then brings it to his or her mouth. Or that an adult accidentally drops a spoon on the floor while setting the table and picks it back up without cleaning it. It might at first seem unlikely that the child or adult might be infected by a virus originally found on the sidewalk, and yet this happens all the time.

Of course, adopting special footwear or paper shoe covers around the house is going a step too far, so to speak, but we can nonetheless draw inspiration from this hospital practice. Just take a look around the world at all the cultures in which taking one's shoes off when entering a house is a standard act of courtesy, synonymous with respect for the host. It is also a very easy hygienic measure to adopt. Too often in the Western world, we place our trust in doormats, which, by dint of having dirt scraped onto them from many a shoe, are breeding grounds for germs. By wiping our feet—an absurd practice, in terms of hygiene—we actually recover the germs of whoever was there before us, which have had, in the intervening time and perhaps dampness, a chance to multiply. To maintain a healthier living environment with fewer bacteria and viruses, make it habit to take off your shoes before entering someone else's home, and ask guests to do the same in your own.

Moving from the floor to countertops and other surfaces, let's stop and sniff the flowers for a moment. There's nothing like a bouquet of fresh flowers to brighten up a room. Rules for preventing infections recommend that a few drops of bleach be placed in vases containing cut flowers. This is an exceedingly simple thing to do, and full of good sense. Microbes develop easily in stagnant water. All you have to do is glance at a pond to see the same principle at work as in a petri dish. In your own home and garden, you are advised not to let water stand, whether in a vase or a backyard pond, without being replaced.

Taking hospital practices as a model and working backward from there provides many possible ways of revising the rules of daily hygiene for greater effectiveness. To revisit the subject of hand washing, for example: Several studies have shown the influence of clean hands on the prevention of nosocomial infections. Hands should not only be washed before each meal and after every trip to the bathroom, but also upon returning home from any outing, to avoid bringing germs from outside back into the house. This hygienic habit has proved tremendously effective in the struggle against the transmission of countless salmonella and staphylococcus infections.

Dangers from Within:
Indoor Pollution

The man who has begun to live more seriously within begins to live more simply without.
                                        —ERNEST HEMINGWAY

Not long ago, a young woman who had been working for several days in a room of newly varnished parquet flooring suddenly had a violent asthma attack, which she did not survive. The culprit behind this brutal death? Formaldehyde, a gas given off by the varnishing product. This compound can be found everywhere in the confined spaces of our living quarters, in amounts that, while admittedly minuscule, can be enough to cause respiratory problems over longer periods of time. Formaldehyde and other toxic substances can be found in the places where we live, and constitute a veritable source of pollution.

We hear talk of pollution with regard to the world outside all the time. Air quality is the object of constant analysis in the media, and the exact amounts of common pollutants are monitored daily. However, the greatest risks are not only outdoors, but inside as well.

Pollution on Every Level

Every recent study has pointed out that the air in our homes is polluted by many chemical products. Tobacco smoke was once a major pollutant, but today it is far from being the only poisonous substance on a long list that includes cleaning supplies, furniture polish, deodorizers, scented fresheners, and even certain adhesives used in particleboard or wallpaper.

In practical terms, these products release chemical compounds that we breathe in every day: formaldehyde, glycol ethers, benzene, terpenes—not to mention the sadly infamous asbestos, which secretes microfibers, invisible to the naked eye but far from harmless. Hundreds of people have been killed by pleural mesothelioma (a cancer of the lungs' protective lining) caused by asbestos.

For want of sufficient circulation, interior air quickly turns into a cocktail of toxic products that can cause colds—which have doubled in number over the past decade—or asthma. The number of asthma-related deaths has risen by 44 percent in the same period. To a lesser degree, interior pollution can cause eye and nose irritation, sore throat, headaches, and fatigue.

Today, we still lack studies to evaluate the impact of these various compounds on our health. As with cigarettes and lung cancer, many years may go by before symptoms appear, and even then, the exact causes are not easy to establish. Moreover, genetic differences among individuals play a very large part: we were not all created equal with regard to tolerance and susceptibility.

It's important to limit the use of toxic cleaning products and construction materials. Denmark, a pioneer in air quality control, recently created an Indoor Climate Labeling Scheme, which gives manufacturers the right to label safe materials for building and beautifying homes, thereby providing companies with the incentive to produce healthier goods. The Environmental Protection Agency in the United States, following a similar logic, classes materials according to their VOC (volatile organic compound) content.

Little Extras That Don't Add Up

In discussing "new" rules of hygiene, we necessarily call into question a few older practices and received ideas, sometimes unfounded, as well as the supposedly efficient products and so-called discoveries that have been developed on the basis of these practices.

Let's start by examining alcohol's capacity to disinfect hands. It should be known that this substance loses some of its decontaminating power in the presence of organic material. Dousing your hands in alcohol is only useful if there's no visible dirt on them. If there is, you should wash your hands first with soap and water, then use an antiseptic sanitizer, which usually takes the form of a hydroalcoholic solution that should not in any way take the place of hand washing. Alcohol-based hand sanitizers are considered supplementary and are useful only in certain specific situations, such as in dentists' offices.

In general, only what is already clean should be disinfected and sterilized. This principle also applies when cleaning house. The most common cleaning error consists in skipping soap and water and using a powerful disinfectant. Since microorganisms thrive in dust and organic residue, it's pointless to spray even a very powerful disinfectant on a spot of dried, solidified food: the dried droplet must first be scrubbed away, and then the area wiped down with disinfectant. In short, scrubbing is the simplest and most effective thing we can do.

Antibacterial wipes, which are quite the fashion right now, do not sufficiently cleanse dirty surfaces, nor do they disinfect spots and stains. They can be used to supplement effective cleaning but cannot take its place.

Another often-seen, but ultimately useless, impulse is to increase the amount of cleaning product used for greater effectiveness. Know that the amount prescribed on the label is calculated for optimal results. Using a larger quantity will only leave a deposit on surfaces without affecting the level of overall cleanliness in the least. Worse yet, using too much increases the risk of toxicity: respiratory irritation, allergies . . . a whole new can of worms!

Using several different disinfecting products simultaneously can also prove dangerous. Using bleach and an ammonia-based product together, for example, triggers a chemical reaction that produces chlorine gas, which is highly

toxic. In the same way, mixing pure ammonia with products containing hypochloric acid causes the formation of
chloramine, a respiratory irritant. Another handy warning:
mixing bleach with acidic products such as descalers causes
the formation of dichlorine, which can cause coughing
and a sensation of respiratory burning.

Hygiene at Home

> When the sun enters your home, it enters your heart
> a little as well.
>
> —LE CORBUSIER

Air quality in the places where we live and work is a fundamental element of good health that remains, even today, too often neglected, provoking any number of conditions, from the serious to the benign—conditions that are, above all, preventable with a few simple habits. Too many families spend all year on antibiotics because of chronic ear, nose, throat, or respiratory infections that can be avoided. The culprit? Dampness in the home. As we've already learned, germs love water, the ideal milieu for proliferation. I've compared still ponds in the countryside to overgrown petri dishes: Who would think for a minute to bathe in such filth? Well, damp spots in a room are comparable to small ponds scattered all about, fostering constant bacterial growth! The problem is that they're often overlooked.

Dampness: A Health Hazard

The sources of dampness may be difficult to detect. Water can infiltrate a house in many ways: old leaks, seepage in the walls or roofing, deficiencies of insulation that can cause condensation and thermal bridges. The simple act of living can cause the barometer to rise: Each person produces 0.5 ounces of water vapor per hour simply by breathing, not to mention performing other daily activities such as showering, cooking, washing dishes, and doing laundry, which all together account for an average of five gallons of water a day. If this vapor isn't gotten rid of quickly—for example, through a range hood or open windows—it settles not only on the walls, but also on fabrics and all the furniture, creating multiple sources of potential microbial development, and all without our necessarily knowing any better.*

A Shower of Problems

Many studies support the correlation between the frequency of respiratory diseases and habitats with high levels of humidity. High levels of humidity give rise to many other problems: the spread of bacteria and dust mites, the

---

*Sick building syndrome (SBS) affects people even in buildings that are apparently sanitary and modern within and without. Occupants complain of skin, eye, sensory, and respiratory symptoms, headaches, watery eyes, and colds. Often the air-filtration system is at fault. Improved air quality control would make these troubles vanish.

proliferation of fungi, and the decay of building materials, which leads to the release of toxic compounds. Allergies, indoor pollution, and respiratory problems are all part of the mix.

Year-round exposure aggravates symptoms, since repeated and prolonged contact with various detrimental agents adds up to a significant dose. Molds, of which several hundred species exist, deserve special mention. Dampness provides ideal conditions for their growth. Their vegetative mycelia spread and they release spores into the air, paving the way for infection. With a mold concentration of up to a million spores per gram of dust, mattresses can become a very major health hazard.

Beware of Fungal Spores

With diameters as small as one micron, fungal spores are capable of penetrating the very depths of respiratory pathways, transporting allergens and toxins with potentially disastrous consequences. Many are the illnesses thus caused, among them rhinitis, bronchitis, and asthma. In addition, molds give off something called secondary metabolites, which are compounds not directly involved in the organisms' growth, and which include certain mycotoxins (produced by fungi) and VOCs. Spores can spread these as well. Mycotoxins are known for provoking not only nausea, but cancer.

Some species of mold spores, such as *Stachybotrys chartarum*, or "toxic black mold," produce extremely destructive trichothecene mycotoxins, which cause severe headaches, coughing, and myalgia, or muscle pain. Cases of pulmonary hemorrhaging have been reported in newborns, who are more vulnerable due to their low body weight. A single spot of *S. chartarum* requires testing and removal by specialists, and cannot simply be plastered or painted over.

Other molds secrete toxins that cause inflammations in the bronchial tubes. Still others release VOCs such as acetone, limonene, and methyl ketones. These can give off a characteristic odor, similar to nail-polish remover, indicating contamination. In the case of MVOCs (microbial volatile organic compounds), scientists have shown that tiny quantities are enough to damage your health.

How to Stay Dry?

Following a few simple and logical rules can help combat dampness. Take, first of all, the sun, whose natural drying power can be extended indoors. The sun alleviates mold, so take advantage of it as far as the layout of your home allows: a southern exposure is one example. A south-facing room is a great place for a child, especially one prone to respiratory difficulties. Next, remember the importance of regular and thorough airing-out of rooms after such household activities as laundry or cooking. Lastly, monitor and repair any leaks that occur in the roof or in plumbing within walls and inside cabinetry. In the case of persistent dampness, a technical test of humidity levels and biological analysis of an air sample by a specialized laboratory will permit an accurate assessment, allowing you to take suitable measures.

The Great Outdoors at Home

You can reduce airborne bacteria and other poisonous elements at home by opening the windows as often as possible, in order to refresh indoor air and reduce poisonous elements. This has proved remarkably effective. Even in winter, awareness of the need to conserve energy should not lead us to shut ourselves in so tightly that toxins and microbes build up with the lack of air changes. Insufficient ventilation poses a very real problem. When we know that the average adult breathes 423 cubic feet of air every day—the approximate equivalent of a six-by-six-by-eighteen-foot room—we can quite quickly grasp why working in a closed space is so unhealthy. Our best defense is always to keep the interiors we live and work in well ventilated by circulating the air for at least five minutes morning and night.

Air Purifiers and Ionizers: Useful or Worthless?

In my opinion, these devices deserve a premier place in the ranks of hygiene scams. All the rage for a few years running, they seem attractive, but only on paper. The idea of purifying the indoors is tempting indeed, but the problem is that no standards are in place to guarantee the effectiveness of this kind of equipment. What's more, some models actually constitute sources of pollution: some produce ozone, while others can turn into breeding grounds for biological pollutants (molds, bacteria) that aggravate allergies. Vaporizing essential oils, too, is of no particular interest, hygienically speaking.

Similarly, air purifiers that claim to combat dust-mite allergies are of questionable effectiveness. The reason is quite simple: because dust mite allergens, carried by large particles, don't stay suspended in the air for long, the purifier doesn't catch them. What's more, dead dust mites break up into fine particles that stick to existing dust. If the air in the room isn't churned about by a broom or a cheap vacuum, these remain on the floor until they are stirred up and, unless caught by the purifier, will enter the lungs. All in all, air purifiers are of little interest where strategies for evicting dust mites are concerned—better to stick with the guidelines outlined in chapter 5.

Deadly Gardens

More things grow in a garden than are sown by a
gardener.

—SPANISH PROVERB

Gardening comes highly recommended as a physical
activity. Moving around outdoors, getting closer to nature (the better to understand it), playing one's small part
in a personal ecology: these do the body good as well as the
spirit. However, in order to make this leisure activity truly
healthy, it behooves the gardener to keep in mind a few
dangers related to working outdoors.

Tetanus: Still Dangerous

Contrary to received wisdom, this disease is far from being eradicated, and occurs quite frequently in developing
countries. What has it got to do with gardening? Tetanus
is most often transmitted by spores in the earth, which
make their way into our bodies via wounds caused by working the soil with bare hands. Symptoms begin with trismus,

or "lockjaw": a violent contraction of the jaw muscles. The contraction spreads to the pharynx, and then to the rest of the body. When it reaches the respiratory muscles, it becomes life threatening. A high price to pay for a little leisurely planting—all the more so as tetanus can be quite simply avoided through vaccination.

In general, these immunizations are up-to-date in children but not adults, who all too often forget to go in for boosters once a decade. When was your last tetanus shot? Whether you're a gardener or not, take a peek at your immunization record. It could help prevent some very nasty surprises.

Hantavirus Haunts the Garden

Small garden rodents can be infected by hantaviruses. These are found in their urine or feces, which are then mixed in with the soil, where gardeners risk contamination by breathing them in, though hantaviruses may also enter the body through an open wound.

Once transmitted to humans, the hantavirus first causes flulike symptoms, which quickly escalate into serious kidney failure accompanied by hemorrhagic signs. Two weeks sometimes go by between contamination and the first symptoms. One symptom is fairly strange and often helps with the diagnosis: sudden, acute myopia, or nearsightedness. Prevention consists of eliminating rodents, wearing a mask when working in dusty outdoor locations such as sheds, and wearing gloves.

Legionellosis in Every Flowerpot

In June 2000, in Washington State, a forty-six-year-old woman was hospitalized for pneumonia. The patient reported that she had been repotting plants during the ten days before her symptoms began. Tests run on samples from the patient allowed doctors to identify the germ found in both the potting soil and the compost in her flowerpots: *Legionella longbeachae*.

Other, similar cases have been reported in the United States, some of which have ended in death from pneumonia. Several studies conducted in diverse regions around the world have proved beyond a doubt that potting soil and compost contain a great number of infectious agents, in particular the genus of bacteria *Legionellas*. In Japan, an analysis of seventeen samples showed the presence of thirty-one different strains of *Legionella*.

Even if all we have are a few blooms in a window planter, we are exposing ourselves to considerable risk. Here, as before, the preventive measure is obvious: wear gloves when handling potting soil. Consider wetting the soil before transferring it, in order to limit the amount of dust floating around in the air.

Sandboxes: Playground Menaces

Our own backyards, decks, porches, and balcony planters aren't the only places where danger of contamination by pathogenic agents resides: public outdoor facilities also present certain risks. Sandboxes are beloved by children but also by dogs, cats, and pigeons. Signs and fences are only so effective in dissuading animals from leaving excrement in sandboxes—pigeons, in particular, pay them no mind! As a result, many parasites can be found in the sand—notably parasites of the *Toxocara* family, including dog or cat round-worms, which cause toxocariasis.

Toxocara roundworms infect the digestive tracts of 45 per-cent of cats and dogs under a year old. The ingestion of con-taminated sand by a child can lead to transmission. Swallowing this parasite's eggs allows them to hatch into larvae in the intestines. Diagnosis is made by observing an increase in certain blood cells—eosinophils and white corpuscles—as well as the presence of the antigen for the disease. The fever and other symptoms go away as the dis-ease runs its course.

In most cases, that is. In others, such severe complica-tions can arise as visceral larva migrans, infections due to immature migrating larvae ousted by the liver's destruc-tion of larvae. Examinations will show a swollen liver and spleen. The victim will, moreover, be irritable and fever-ish, with a loss of appetite. Boys and girls from ages one to five are the most often affected.

Modern medicine has this type of pathology well under control, but a better solution is to avoid it altogether. Accord-ing to *Allergy: European Journal of Allergy and Clinical Im-munology*, the parasite *Toxocara* can be found, on average, in one out of four sandboxes. A reasonable response to this would be to rethink the design of the sandbox itself. Site selection and some form of drainage or runoff system are key elements, as is the quality of the sand itself (granite, quartz, and certain other crushed sands should be avoided). Next, proper upkeep is essential: manual cleaning, sifting, and disinfection via different procedures—steaming at 284 degrees Fahrenheit, mechanical filtration, or microwave—have proved to noticeably decrease the presence of parasites.

PART IV

HYGIENE AND LIFESTYLE

"Purity and impurity are personal; no person can purify another," said Buddha. In today's globalized world, where exchanges and transactions of every sort occur and multiply at increasing rates, these words remind us that there are limits to what can be shared. Far from taking a detour into spirituality, this next part will discuss quite concretely what rules of hygiene individuals can follow to share good times, rather than germs, with friends and loved ones.

A How-to of Personal Hygiene

Even the best shower won't wash away all your blues.
—DANIEL PENNAC

In 1926, the *Little Illustrated Larousse* encyclopedia accompanied its definition of the word *hygiene* with the following advice: "Good skin care includes inuring your skin to cold by washing it daily with ice water; taking a hot bath once a week in every season maintains good health and prevents chills." In our age of heated towel racks, hot running water, and balneotherapy at home, the quaintness of such counsel brings a smile. It also reminds us that standard practices in personal hygiene are constantly evolving. Life today entails new rules.

Bath or Shower?

The answer is clear from a hygienic as well as an ecological point of view: showers are preferable to baths. Baths use up an enormous amount of water but don't leave us any cleaner. They encourage soaking, and the longer they last, the more germs there are, frolicking about. The thin gray film that settles on the inside of the bathtub after the water drains away gives us some idea of what a petri dish we've been sitting in. A bath should be preceded or followed by a shower and a good soaping. Beware, also, of excessively hot baths, as they may cause a drop in blood pressure. All this, in any case, proves the Japanese right: baths are not made for cleaning the body.

Household showers, on the other hand, came into this world as a direct result of hydrotherapy, originally used in spas. Their history begins with the English invention of the tub in which one stood upright and plunged a sponge into the water before squeezing it out above one's head. Little by little, basins with curtains to minimize splashing, and then the showerhead, made their appearance in rudimentary forms. With the fancy contemporary systems of multiple adjustable nozzles, the shower returns to something like its roots in hydrotherapy, where its purpose was to provide full body massage and promote skin circulation. No longer dedicated solely to hygiene, the shower has become a part of healthy living in general, firmly establishing its supremacy over the bath.

Morning or Night?

Ideally, one should shower twice a day, but conserving water—a very fragile and vital resource—is a necessity in our day and age. Many of us shower in the morning, and that serves us quite well, but sometimes doing it again at night can prove necessary, especially when we take into account the possible contamination our bodies have undergone in the course of a normal workday. In cases where professional activities expose people to microbial or chemical agents, it's better to take a shower while still at work or at a gym, rather than track such contaminants into one's home. Cases have been reported where people who worked with lead and returned directly home contaminated their children. This might have been averted with a shower and a change of clothes at the workplace.

In situations like these, showering in the evening becomes necessary. Beware, however, of hot baths at night. Although relaxing, they do not encourage sleep. Toward bedtime, anything that raises the body's temperature promotes wakefulness. At night, body temperature should start slowly decreasing toward its lowest level, around 3AM.

From Head to Toes, or Toes on Up?

Where should we start when washing ourselves? The ergonomics of hygiene can be surprising, especially when we think back on just who taught us to wash ourselves the way we do. There are surely as many ways to go about it as there are people in the world. It's often been a source of amusement for me to poll the people around me on the order in which they prefer to wash themselves, just to hear the variety of responses and the reasons behind them, which are governed by every principle except logic.

Yet logic is what matters here. Ergonomics and common sense tell us to go with the flow—that is, of water from head to toes—so that the suds can take dirt and germs with them as they run down our bodies. Better to wash with plain soap and water than a glove, washcloth, or pouf, unless you plan to change these after every use.

Let me add here that only the exteriors of genitalia should be washed. Modern medicine advises against daily vaginal douches except in the case of specific infections. Most soaps are too harsh for women to use in intimate washing. The sensitive mucous membranes of this part of the anatomy provide natural protection. The vagina is a self-cleansing body part.

A Clean, Well-Lighted Toilet Seat

The vast majority of toilets, public or private, are equipped with a flush mechanism, which leads us to the work of Professors Gerba and Willis in the United States. They have shown that the moment someone pushes down on that handle, the resulting flush produces an aerosol effect that sprays germs all over the room. Their study, based on an analysis of initially sterile surfaces (wall tiles in particular), clearly points out the viruses and bacteria colonies spread by projected moisture.

Professor Gerba pursued his research on the aerosol effect at greater length, notably by establishing that pathogenic agents were left pirouetting in the air for two hours after an initial flush and could be found on many nearby surfaces, including toilet paper awaiting the next user. In addition, he drew attention to the link between inhaling these germs and certain respiratory diseases.

Another study, conducted in Japan on 5,854 subjects by Professor Ueda, also demonstrated the correlation between contamination rates from *Helicobacter pylori* and flushing. Still other research indicates that one in every three Americans flushes while seated—an act which, any disagreeable moisture aside, heightens the risk of infection.

The necessary preventive measure is obvious: lower the toilet seat lid before flushing. Additionally, in order to avoid all recontamination, Gerba recommends using a paper towel to shut off faucets and to open doors after hand washing.

This might seem excessive, but facts from a recent American study on public bathrooms reveal even more unusual behavior:

- 48 percent of women cover toilet seats with toilet paper.
- 15 percent of Americans use paper towels to turn faucet knobs.
- 8 percent use *their feet* to flush.

- 2 percent use their wrist or elbow to advance the paper towel roll.

No point in going that far: the simple measures outlined in this chapter will suffice to limit risks of infection considerably.

Skin Deep

We are all tattooed in our cradles with the beliefs of our tribe; the record may seem superficial, but it is indelible.

—OLIVER WENDELL HOLMES JR.

L ove 'em or loathe 'em, tattoos and piercings have risen sharply in popularity these last few years. Such ornamentation, once relatively marginal, now seems almost conventional. However, standards and practices have not kept up: those providing tattoos and piercings are often considered artists rather than technicians and, perhaps as a result, do not always conform to sanitary regulations.

Yet the procedures involved are far from safe. Getting a piercing or a tattoo under the wrong circumstances can have serious consequences. Recent publications highlight the risks associated with these practices: possible contraction of viral hepatitis B and C, as well as microbial infection (staphylococcal, streptococcal, and pyocyaneous). The infectious mechanism can have many possible origins: poorly sterilized materials, tainted blood, contamination by the customer's skin itself if poorly disinfected before the act.

It is difficult to understand the reasons for legislative passivity in the face of such risks. In order to give a simple injection, nurses must be registered by the state after three years of study; how is it that no qualifications are required to administer a tattoo or a piercing, procedures often more complicated than an inoculation? Moreover, with piercings, anatomical ignorance on the artist's part can result in implants in areas close to nerve endings or blood vessels.

Tattoo and piercing artists are certainly not all to be put in the same boat: if some are unscrupulous, others practice their profession in laudable conditions, inform their customers of the risks they run, and refuse to perform procedures they deem dangerous. However, in the absence of regulation, the consumer has no guarantees.

A Study That Gets Under the Skin

A particularly interesting study was performed on eight piercing and tattoo parlors in the Hérault province of southeastern France, in order to evaluate the exact risks to which customers were subjected. The results speak for themselves.

First, the tattoo artists all used tattoo guns. In these devices, an ink tube attaches to a needle in direct contact with the skin. Gun and needle are disposable, single-use items, yet they are typically reused from one client to the next. The needles, ordered in boxes of a thousand, are nonsterile.

Second, ink of unknown composition, came in unlabeled bottles, to each tattoo parlor from its own provider. This gives some cause for alarm, since cases of poisoning have occurred when inks used in processed-food packaging have simply come into contact with the skin. Such inks have been banned, but who knows what ingredients might be in the ink used for tattoos? Here again, we have a glaring lack of regulation.

The study of tattoo parlors did, however, show that some artists were aware of such risks as hepatitis and AIDS. Four owners had been inoculated against hepatitis B, and two regularly underwent AIDS screening. All wore gloves when working, but more to keep from getting ink on their hands than out of health considerations.

The bottom line here is that where sterilization was concerned, none of the parlors in the study followed the necessary, indispensable steps of decontamination, cleaning, and packaging preparatory to sterilization itself. In most cases, some display of sterilization was made, giving the client a false sense of security. Four tattoo parlors used Poupinel dry-heat sterilizers, but observed neither the minimum required times nor temperatures.

Worse yet, none of the practitioners in the study had an autoclave, a steam-pressure device essential for sterilizing medical instruments. Should it be any surprise that among the biological samples taken during the study, eleven were nonsterile?

No two ways about it: the results of this study are enough to give one goose bumps. From the ink tubes of tattoo guns whose exudations enter into contact with skin and blood from multiple customers during the tattooing process, to body rings that present the risk of infection if not properly sterilized before insertion, the microbiological hazards are significant.

Dangerous Beauty

Tattoos and piercings are far from having a monopoly on such dangers. Cosmetic dermapigmentation, to which some women resort for a permanently made-up look, also demands flawless sanitary practices. Even jewelers offering ear piercings are not above reproach. A number of them use "piercing guns" to put in earrings. The bases of such devices are sullied with each use, becoming carriers of infection for the next client if no strict and effective decontamination is practiced.

Wouldn't it be simpler and safer for everyone if specific standards of sterilization were imposed? How much longer must we tolerate "artists" performing procedures on customers' bodies in contempt of the most basic rules of medical hygiene? While waiting for the law to change, I can only call on everyone to be vigilant and ask those wishing to be tattooed or pierced to think twice. In any case, use very strict standards when selecting a tattoo or piercing parlor, and do not hesitate to consult a doctor if you experience any discomfort after the procedure.

Hair and Nail Salons

At first, this might seem a silly thought, but it is, in fact, quite a reasonable one. Imagine that you are to have an operation. An hour before going into surgery, you watch, from behind a one-way mirror, orderlies prepare the room. The surgeon has just finished up with the preceding patient and decides to clean, all by himself, the stained instruments he'll be using on you next. Briskly, with a cotton ball dunked in some vague disinfecting product, he swabs down the scissors and the scalpels, passes them quickly through the blue glow from a box-like device, and just like that, he's done: everything is ready for you, the next patient. You'd be offended if you saw as much. And yet that's exactly what happens at hair and nail salons. The correct reaction to such a display would be to flee the scene at top speed, for if you were to examine the instruments under a microscope, you'd see them still covered, to your great fright, in numerous viruses and bacteria.

That many serious diseases such as hepatitis and AIDS are transmitted through the blood is well known. When an instrument has been in contact with someone's blood, it must be properly sterilized. At hair or nail salons, during a quick trim or a manicure, tiny cuts are commonplace. A little bloodletting, and it's over. If the same minor inconvenience has befallen one of the customers before you, it's as if you were being operated on by a surgeon using contaminated instruments: without even knowing it, you run the risk of a potentially dangerous infectious transmission.

Think back to how your stylist, pedicurist, or manicurist goes about his or her business. Some, aware of the potential dangers, sterilize their instruments impeccably between clients. Others, less thorough, merely go through the motions. Don't hesitate to ask questions in order to inform yourself better. Respect for hygiene conditions is essential in these environments, for the sake of clients as well as the professionals, who expose themselves to the same risks. AIDS and hepatitis can indeed be passed on in such a context.

Just as we've seen with tattoos and piercings, certain practices at salons turn out to be ineffective displays. To point out just one: dipping instruments in alcohol and setting them alight. The resulting temperature is far from sufficient, and the instruments are in no way sterilized. Admittedly, fire is the symbol of purification and alcohol of disinfection, but this quick procedure is of no real use. Let me repeat: Instruments must be sterilized according to the rules. Sterilization by steam pressure in an autoclave is, to date, the most effective, reliable, and easy-to-use method. If an autoclave is unavailable, a long soak (at least fifteen minutes) in a powerful disinfectant (combining bactericide, virucide, fungicide, and sporicide) is called for.

The goal of sterilization is to completely eliminate all germs present on an object, whether pathogenic or not. In theory, sterility as a state is defined by the total absence of bacteria. In reality, this state is impossible to achieve. By convention, the sterility threshold is set at one chance in a million of finding an active germ after sterilization. Once decontaminated, instruments can be kept in sterile condition for several months if correctly packaged.

Skin Preparations for Tanning

A few years ago, there appeared on the market oral supplements that, according to their manufacturers, allowed users to prepare their skin for exposure to the sun. At first glance a godsend for people who burn easily, the marketing campaign led people to believe that these pills could reduce the risk of skin cancer. In fact, a large number of people believe, mistakenly, that artificial UV light, tanning creams, and tanning pills actually ready the skin for the sun's assault, protecting them from cancer and the signs of premature aging.

This could not be further from the truth: the risk remains the same despite these treatments, except in rare, very specific cases of medical care.* In all other instances,

---

*We may, for example, cite PUVA therapy sessions conducted by a dermatologist as part of a preventive treatment for benign summer light eruption (BSLE), a condition that manifests itself as skin eruptions after exposure to the sun.

the connection between sun exposure and skin cancer, as well as premature aging, has been clearly established. Even so, the desire to come back from vacation with a nice tan, so long synonymous with good health, moves many people to prolong their exposure to UV rays, thereby inviting serious damage to their health.

Faced with the dangers of the sun, vigilance is a must. This is even truer in the mountains, where the intensity of the sun's rays increases by 20 percent with every three-thousand-foot increase in elevation. Caution should not be confined to summertime alone: spring or fall weekends can easily cause sunburn as well. When sunburn occurs repeatedly, even from limited exposure to sunlight, it may be due to a side effect from medication, or certain illnesses, and one should see a doctor about it.

Apart from being painful and unsightly, sunburn has harmful effects at the biological level. Exposure to sunlight causes a reaction at the DNA level that shows up as photoderived products and free radicals. These lead to the deterioration of cellular membranes as well as conjunctival tissue.

What's more, the link between skin cancer and exposure to UV radiation has been demonstrated beyond a doubt. There are two types of ultraviolet rays: UVA which, thanks to a photochemical reaction, causes rapid but short-lived tanning, and UVB, which results in a slower but longer-lasting tan. Both can give rise to skin cancer.

The cumulative effect of exposure to UV rays over a period of many dozens of years increases the danger. This important fact underlines the necessity of effective solar protection from childhood onward. Clothes are a good place to start, especially broad-brimmed hats. Know that the thicker an article of clothing is and the darker its color, the better defense it offers. A white cotton T-shirt lets through up to 20 percent of UV rays and up to 50 percent if wet. The same shirt in black is much less easily penetrated by solar radiation.

As for sunscreens and other sun products, bear in mind that none provide complete protection against UV rays, not even the ones that claim to do so. Spending hours in the sun, believing yourself encased in sunscreen as if in a suit of armor, amounts to a terrible misconception, especially if you don't take care to reapply the product at least every two hours.

How much do we really know about sun protection products and how they're tested? To start, lotions or sprays have two kinds of filters, physical and chemical, often combined in the same product.

Physical filters are mineral pigments that reflect and disperse UV rays. They act on the surface, without penetrating the skin, where they would no longer be effective. Chemical filters, on the other hand (often called UVA and UVB filters, depending on the kind of radiation they screen out), absorb UV radiation by transforming energy-rich short-wavelength rays into less-powerful long-wavelength rays. This conversion takes place inside the skin, once the sunscreen has been well absorbed. In order to be fully effective, sunscreen should be applied thirty minutes before exposure to the sun—which is all too rarely done.

And so we come to the index of protectiveness specified on product labels. SPF, or sun protection factor, indicates the possible duration of exposure to the sun before the appearance of an erythema, or reddening. In order to calculate this duration, researchers apply two milligrams of the product per square centimeter of skin, which comes to about one to one and a half ounces of lotion for an adult body. In practice, how many of us use this much? Let's not kid ourselves: practically no one ever uses this dose. As a direct consequence, the protection factor is reduced by half or even three-quarters. A product that purports to have an SPF of 20 corresponds, in reality, to a protective index of 5 to 10 if you don't apply it in sufficient quantities. Pay attention, also, to products claiming to be waterproof or water-resistant: these should be reapplied, on average, once every two swims, as they do not remain "resistant" forever.

Ultimately, a lotion claiming maximum protection is a good idea, but doesn't constitute a total barrier against the sun. The most effective defense is still a parasol, a hat, and sunglasses, and remaining indoors during peak sunlight hours. People more susceptible to sunburn, such as children or pregnant women, must adhere all the more strictly to these measures, as the latter run the risk of a melasma or "mask of pregnancy" dark brown patches that appear on the face (especially cheeks, forehead, and temples). It's important not to confuse products that purport to "prepare" the skin but have, in actuality, only a cosmetic effect, with those that offer a real protective barrier.

Being Selfish About Hygiene

Lend yourself to others, but give yourself only to yourself.

—MONTAIGNE

As we've seen several times now, germs need a carrier to spread from person to person, be it saliva, blood, hands, or the paraphernalia of daily life. To check the needless spread of germs and pests, we must sometimes be selfish, neither lending nor swapping certain personal items. Hats, combs, headbands, barrettes, and hairbrushes are strictly for the use of a single person only, lest lice, fleas, ticks, crabs, or ringworms take advantage of the vehicle to find a new host.

To prevent contamination of the bloodstream—a greater danger still—personal objects possibly bearing traces of blood (razors, nail clippers, makeup and depilatory applicators, toothbrushes) must not be shared. In the case of herpes, lipstick, lip gloss, and lip balm must absolutely not be shared, not even by best friends. Such carriers spread the virus quite easily. Toothbrushes are associated with specific additional risks that deserve attention.

The Terrible Toothbrush

An American study published in July 2004 on the toothbrush revealed this everyday object to be an unbelievably effective medium for spreading germs. First, the oral cavity already contains many germs, and second, germs need two things to grow: moisture and time. A toothbrush, quickly rinsed after brushing, is a hotbed of bacterial activity par excellence in which streptococcus, staphylococcus, herpes, and the flu virus readily proliferate. Toothbrushes are even capable of transmitting such serious viral pathologies as hepatitis among people within a single household. The virus can survive for up to a week on bristles.

Besides never lending out your toothbrush, remember to change it as a rule after colds and infections of the nose or throat. Many people unknowingly reexpose themselves to infection when they brush their teeth, because their own germs have multiplied on their toothbrushes between uses.

Next, avoid keeping your toothbrush in a moist, dark bathroom cabinet; this encourages bacterial growth. Ideally, a toothbrush should be kept near a window or in a dry, well-ventilated area. A little tip: shake the water from the bristles and dry it with a disposable napkin. Rid of its moisture, a toothbrush is no longer an ideal place for germs.

Last but not least, get a new toothbrush every month!

This might seem excessive to some people, especially in terms of budget. But from the point of view of hygiene, better to buy a cheaper model and replace it more often than the most expensive kind and keep it for six months: whatever its price, a toothbrush turns into a veritable bacterial reservoir after about five weeks of steady use.

To Each His Own Towel

Proper hygiene requires us neither to share toothbrushes nor towels, not even with our family members. Towels can pass on many sexually transmitted diseases, mycoses, bacterial infections, and parasites, especially if they remain damp several days at a time. Again, the duo of warmth and dampness promotes microbial proliferation. If the body parts of the person who used the towel before you were less than immaculate, this should give you pause.

Upon stepping out of the shower, dry yourself thoroughly with a clean towel. Towels should be thought of as tissues—for use by a single individual only—as germs love to multiply on them. When drying between the legs, dry the front first and then the rear, and not the other way around, in order to avoid contaminating the genitals and the urinary tract with anal bacteria—a common error, often the source of cystitis or vaginitis.

Hang towels out to dry after each use. Never ball damp towels up and toss them into a laundry basket or, worse yet, a corner of the room. Change towels at least once a week and above all: keep them to yourself!

Cell Phones: A Hive of Bacteria

American scientists have studied the presence of germs on cell phones in great detail. Their research has demonstrated an average of eleven thousand microbes per square inch on phone surfaces. How can such a figure be explained? First, by the microdroplets we spray on the receiver when speaking. Also, due to the fact these devices rarely get cleaned, especially the less accessible parts.

A good habit to develop would be to avoid borrowing other people's phones and to lend your own out as little as possible. In addition, clean the receiver every morning with a moist towelette, especially when suffering from a cold, a throat infection, or the flu. These two protective measures will help limit the risk of spreading disease to those close to you, but also of recontaminating yourself with your own germs, which can lead to protracted illness.

Throw Out Those Handkerchiefs!

Our noses are our bodies' first line of microbial filters. Given that there are almost two hundred extremely contagious viruses capable of causing the common cold, our noses can't afford to slack off on the job. Luckily, most viruses never make it past the nasal mucous membranes; still, adults suffer on average from two to five colds per year, and children even more. In order to keep these figures from increasing, let's not expose our noses to more pathogens than we have to. That's exactly what we do, however, when we use cloth handkerchiefs.

When you have a cold, you often have to blow your nose and clear out nasal secretions that contain microbes capable of multiplying, especially on the fabric of a handkerchief wadded up in a warm, dark pocket. The next time you use that handkerchief, you expose yourself to viruses more virulent and numerous than before. Your cold has every chance of dragging on for weeks as a result. Let's not even talk about the risks involved should you lend your handkerchief to someone else. Use paper tissues, which are very hygienic so long as they're disposed of immediately after use. And don't forget to cover your nose and mouth when sneezing or coughing: droplets of saliva can hit speeds of up to 105 miles per hour!

Can the Cold Carry Germs?

How many generations have been raised on the words: "Cover up, or you'll catch cold!"? Let's take a minute to banish the myth associating the *cold* itself with the onset of illness. No scientific evidence supports this claim. While it is true that low temperatures weaken our bodies and make us more vulnerable to infections, cold air does not carry any more germs, or especially encourage their spread—unlike contaminated individuals who neglect the basic rules of hygiene.

Dirty Kisses

Among the viruses transmissible by kissing is oral herpes. The initial transmission often goes unnoticed, and symptoms only manifest themselves in 20 percent of cases. The subject complains of inflammation of the gums and mouth, accompanied by painful blisters, swelling of the submaxillary (or throat) glands, and fever. Most people affected experience recurrence in the form of blisters along the lips. Humans are the only known reservoirs for this virus.

Another organism is the Epstein-Barr virus, which causes infectious mononucleosis, a common illness whose symptoms include fever, throat infection, glandular swelling, and enlargement of the spleen. Kissing is a classic means of passing it on, hence the name, the "kissing disease." This may explain why 80 percent of those afflicted are between eighteen and twenty-five years of age, a time of frequent romantic encounters. The recurrence of mononucleosis is generally benign.

Other illnesses, such as mumps, may also be transmitted by saliva. It is important to limit direct contact with others throughout the entire period of contagion, when you or they are symptomatic of herpes or another viral infection. Correct hygiene entails not sharing towels, drinking glasses, or clothing, as well as wiping up after yourself after a meal and washing up thoroughly. Dishes should be washed at a minimum temperature of 120 degrees Fahrenheit.

Teeth and Bacteria

I'm losing my teeth, I'm dying one detail at a time.
—VOLTAIRE

B rushing your teeth is a regular daily activity. However, it isn't always enough to ensure perfect oral hygiene. It so happens that a simple oral infection can sometimes have disastrous, even life-threatening consequences for one's health.

From Toothaches to Brain Abscesses

A dental focus of infection constitutes a reserve for germs, which can sporadically migrate—over weeks, months, or even years—toward heart valves. Pyorrhea alveolaris (periodontitis), and erythematous stomatitis (mouth ulcers) are local complications with one thing in common: the pain they cause, which, fortunately, prompts sufferers to prioritize a trip to the dentist. In other cases, persistent bad breath may be behind the visit. The dentist then discovers cavities or an attack under way on the periodontium, bleeding gums and all, which he or she can treat before troubles of another sort rear their heads. For if these dental problems go untreated, or arise without causing the subject excessive discomfort, they can insidiously spread microbes throughout the body. What begins as a dental infection colonizes neighboring anatomical areas, creating new infected zones that, in their turn, go on to infect other areas.

Various problems may manifest themselves, from swollen glands in the neck region to chronic ear, nose, and throat infections, all stemming from a tooth in poor shape from which germs regularly migrate. Persistent otitis (ear infection), sinusitis, throat infection, pharyngitis (sore throat), or laryngitis should cause you to seek out a dental exam. Although any antibiotics prescribed for these conditions may prove effective for a short while, a few weeks later, the infected tooth will have sent out more germs, provoking a recurrence. The only way to put an end to such relapses is to address the problem at its source.

Given time, complications even more severe can occur: Septic metastases can form and be carried by the blood, causing lung infections and even brain abscesses. Every year, quite a few patients are hospitalized for unexplained fevers, or rushed to intensive care for life-threatening septicemia, because of dental infections left uncared for! The risk of complications is heightened for people who do not maintain strict oral hygiene habits. These can include people, such as diabetics or the HIV-positive, whose immune defenses have already been weakened. Their regular medical checkups must include dental exams. But other people turn out to be at risk as well, often without their knowing it. The danger is quite real, for it threatens the heart.

Teeth and Endocarditis

Every year, thousands of people are victims of endocarditis, otherwise known as an inflammation of the inner layer of the heart (endocardium), which affects the heart valves and has a mortality rate ranging from 20 to 30 percent. Subjects fall into two categories. The first know they have a narrowed valve or mitral insufficiency. They usually have regular appointments with a cardiologist, who will recommend regular dental checkups. Moreover, some preventive treatment will have been prescribed: for instance, antibiotics to be taken before dental exams, with a view to warding off possible infection.

For this first category of patients, the risks are relatively limited—but not for the second, who suffer unawares from heart-valve trouble. Their regular physicians might have noticed, or even commented on, a tiny and unserious heart murmur—or have noticed nothing at all. A heart valve with even the smallest of lesions is an environment favorable to microbes. Spreading from a dental focus of infection, they are likely to gather on the valve, with catastrophic consequences: the destruction, ulceration, and perforation of cardiac tissue. At this point the patient will complain of different symptoms such as unexplained fevers or abnormal breathlessness. Diagnosis will find the culprit: often a streptococcus of oral origin. According to the seriousness of the damage done to the valve, the treatment can run from basic antibiotics to surgery for prosthetic replacement of the affected area. In other words, one runs the risk, by not going to the dentist, of winding up in the operating room instead for open-heart surgery.

A Double Dose of Prevention

Open-heart surgery is, to say the least, a procedure that is far from unintrusive. In order to ward off its possibility, we must step up our preventive efforts in two directions: oral hygiene and cardiovascular follow-up care. I'm constantly astonished to see that many people pay more attention to their cars than to their teeth or their hearts. The slightest irregular sound under the hood and they're off to the mechanic. They follow the manufacturer's recommended service guidelines to the letter and check the pressure in their tires quite conscientiously. If they paid as much attention to their blood pressure, they'd surely be able to catch hypertension before it could do any harm. And if they checked their cholesterol as often as they did their oil, they might catch atheromatous plaques (fatty degeneration of the arteries) and reduce the chances of heart attacks and hemiplegia (partial paralysis) by treating them. With this in mind, a visit to the cardiologist every five years becomes a necessity—think of it as an engine checkup—in addition to a yearly trip to the dentist, to monitor potential infections. These habits are the first step on a solid preventive course—provided, of course, that oral hygiene is kept up as well.

Toothcare Tips

Brush your teeth with a soft brush twice a day and after sticky treats to reduce acids and prevent germs from developing. Excessive, hard brushing can cause gum recession. In Brazil, everyone keeps a toothbrush and toothpaste at work. You can do the same.

Publicity campaigns in schools and offices urging children and adults to brush after lunch would be a good step. Next, why not have restaurants and cafeterias keep dental hygiene kits on hand in their restrooms?

In order for brushing to be effective, you must brush your teeth gently on all sides. Thirty seconds is not enough; brush for two to three minutes. Floss at least once a day to get rid of any remaining food particles, and remember to change your toothbrush often.

PART V

GERMS UNDER SURVEILLANCE

We have seen how adopting new personal hygiene habits can help defend us against certain diseases and improve our overall quality of life. The concept of hygiene must now be applied on a much vaster scale, to combat the threats of viruses proliferating planetwide. The scientific community has its eyes on legionellosis, Ebola, H5N1, and other new dangers that represent potential threats to hundreds of millions of people. What, realistically, have we to fear—and what can we do to protect ourselves?

Legions of *Legionella*

Hot water does not forget that it was once cold.
—AFRICAN PROVERB

In 1976, members of the American Legion, a veterans association, gathered for the American Bicentennial convention in a Philadelphia hotel. Shortly thereafter, some of them fell victim to a serious and then-unidentified pneumonia. It was discovered that they had all been infected by the same bacteria, which was dubbed Legionella. It is quite common in many environments, especially in water between 68 and 122 degrees Fahrenheit, where it multiplies rapidly. It proliferates in hot-water tanks, air-conditioning cooling towers, spas, and fountains.

Every Breath You Take

Legionella is always spread in the same way—not from person to person, but by an intermediary that produces a spray or aerosol effect. This may be as simple as a showerhead, a ventilation system, or an air conditioner. Victims breathe in this bacterial spray. After an incubation period from two to ten days, the bacteria cause legionellosis, the symptoms of which include fever and trouble breathing, sometimes degenerating into acute respiratory distress. Treatment consists of antibiotics, sometimes complemented by respiratory assistance.

The foundation of legionellosis prevention lies in the proper upkeep of water and ventilation systems; homeowners and hotel managers alike need to take care of buildup and corrosion, maintain hot water at sufficiently high temperatures, and ensure good recirculation.

Two preventive measures are advised at home. First of all, if your hot water has not been used for some time—for example, while you have been away on vacation—always let it run for a few minutes. Next, if this water comes from a hot-water tank, perform a yearly checkup: there may be deposits of limescale, which promotes the growth of Legionella. It doesn't take much for them to cross the line and become a veritable bacterial legion.

The Ebola Engima

Blood will have blood.
                    —William Shakespeare

The Ebola virus has an important place in the pantheon of the most virulent infectious agents. It first drew attention to itself in 1976, in Sudan and Zaire, and was named after a river in the latter country. Its impact was devastating: 280 dead in Zaire and 150 in Sudan. Another epidemic came about in 2003, claiming still more victims.

A Difficult Epidemic to Fight

One problem lay in the fact that the disease is easily transmitted by human contact. Symptoms present after an incubation period of from four to nine days. Fever, muscle pain, and especially diarrhea and vomiting appear. Next come complications—multiple hemorrhages, kidney failure, and hepatitis can lead to comas and death. The mortality rate runs from 50 to 80 percent, with death most often occurring a week after the first appearance of the symptoms.

Worst of all is the absence of any truly effective medication. Our arsenals remain limited; no vaccine or preventive treatment exists for Ebola. During the 1976 outbreak, the virus took a heavy toll on medical personnel, who were highly exposed to it. Quarantine of infected patients is now imperative during outbreaks. It is essential to limit the number of people in contact with infected subjects to an absolute minimum.

Origins of a Deadly Virus

Hoping to find clues to a cure, scientists have sought the origins of Ebola ever since the virus was first isolated in humans. The virus is most commonly zoonotic—that is, passed from animals to humans. While gorillas were long suspected as transmitters of the virus, a number of arguments now favor the fruit bat.

But an altogether different hypothesis opens up disquieting prospects. Karl Johnson of the University of New Mexico has succeeded in isolating a virus very close in shape to that of Ebola in a small European insect common to yards and gardens. Central African guinea pigs were then found to have Ebola virus antibodies in their blood. The guinea pig, however, is a herbivore. These facts led Johnson to suspect that viruses present in fauna were present in flora as well. Indeed, if plants are sources of Ebola-type viruses, capable of transmitting those viruses to insects or animals, human contamination is an all-too-possible next step. Although this hypothesis has not yet been confirmed, the potential of an outbreak hangs not only over Africa but also Europe.

Clearly, the world cannot afford simply to wait for Johnson's hypothesis to be confirmed or disproved, but must concentrate its efforts in seeking out every last focus of infection in Africa, and hastening research on the virus's origins and possible treatments.

SARS: Can It Happen Again?

Love is like an epidemic. The more one fears it, the higher one's chances of contracting it.

—NICOLAS DE CHAMFORT

In November 2002, the first cases of SARS (severe acute respiratory syndrome) appeared in China, as some readers may remember. On March 12, 2003, the World Health Organization issued a global alert about "a serious and atypical form of pneumonia in Vietnam, Hong Kong, and Canton." On March 22, the antibody was isolated at last, by CDC laboratories in Atlanta. On April 2, the WHO issued a formal advisory against travel to Hong Kong and southern China. The virus, however, continued to spread until July 2003. In total, twenty-eight countries were concerned, eight thousand people were infected, and 774 died. How was this syndrome fought, and what dangers remain today?

A Deadly New Strain

SARS is caused by a coronavirus, of which two strains—HCoV-229E and HCoV-OC43—had previously been reported in humans before 2003. These two bugs were the cause of only benign, even banal respiratory infections and therefore of no particular worry. No discussion of SARS is complete without pointing out the incredible feat of research on the part of laboratories around the world in working to help isolate the new, much more dangerous strain, since identified as SARS-CoV.

Contamination occurs quite simply via saliva from infected subjects, facilitated by the hardiness of the virus itself, which is capable of surviving twenty-four hours on a plastic surface such as an elevator button. The incubation period can last from two to eleven days, after which patients experience flulike symptoms: fever, respiratory difficulty, and digestive troubles. Respiratory complications force a quarter of those afflicted into the ICU, with a mortality rate of around 10 percent, varying by country.

One test, called a PCR (polymerase chain reaction), can detect genetic material from the virus itself in bloody sputum, tissue, or stool samples, but can yield false negatives. Blood serum analysis helps identify the antibodies in case of an epidemic. Chest X-rays are also used. Treatment combines different antibiotics intended to combat secondary respiratory problems, complemented by respiratory assistance where needed.

In order to contain the risks of contamination, drastic measures must be taken: quarantine, in negative-pressure rooms where possible, is imperative, and medical personnel must wear masks, gloves, and protective goggles.

The Dangers Today

The SARS epidemic and ensuing panic amounted to a sort of preview or public dress rehearsal of what an emerging disease might do. It took just one infected man checking in to a Hong Kong hotel on February 21, 2003, for the virus to spread to Singapore and Canada by the twenty-third and twenty-fourth. Assisted by airline travel, an epidemic of this type goes global in a matter of days.

The SARS epidemic was contained through sheer luck. The researchers' amazing performance quickly led to the development of effective treatments, which brought a halt to the virus's spread. The virus, however, has not disappeared, and no vaccine yet exists. In this particular case, medical personnel constituted a third of the victims.

At least one preventive measure exists. Dr. Mark Gendreau of the University of Vermont, along with his coauthor Alexandra Mangili, suggest in their report that changing the onboard air twice as often on a plane would cut the risk of infection by half. The authors' calculations were based on mathematical modeling experiments. In the case of SARS, it seems, we can be relatively at ease—more so, at least, than about other perils.

Avian Influenza: The Real Risks

Can a man be less wise than a bird?

—Confucius

Much has been said about the "bird flu" episode of 2005 to 2006, and much of that is more confusing than informative.

As of 2008, the risk of an outbreak has not been completely dispelled and, although less often in the news, avian flu continues to cause worry. Why did the alert level go gradually red over 2006 and 2007? Why have doctors, the World Health Organization, and other authorities sounded the alarm? Why have millions of people worldwide ordered face masks and stockpiled so many survival kits in case of catastrophe? What are the real dangers facing us today, and how should we defend ourselves?

What's So Frightening About H5N1?

For several dozen years now, episodes of avian flu have regularly arisen without the slightest rumor of pandemic, but with the mid-2004 outbreak in China, things changed radically. A special new variety of the Z genotype, or category, of the H5N1 virus was discovered. Tedious detail aside, this new form of the virus revealed itself to be highly pathogenic, with a very high mortality rate among animals. It spread massively across the globe, going from epizootic—that is, an epidemic affecting a single kind of animal—to panzootic, an epidemic affecting many different species of animals, wild and domestic alike, including cats, ducks, tigers, and geese. As can be expected, the broader its reach throughout the animal kingdom, the more quickly the virus spreads. Moreover, the virus's passing from epizootic to panzootic reveals the added risk that it might mutate again and become transmissible from human to human. This totally new and frightening prospect in part explains the difficulty in managing the crisis. Historical examples—the Spanish flu, for example—are hardly reassuring.

A Preview of Coming Attractions?

The Spanish influenza pandemic of 1918 was so named because Alfonso XIII of Spain caught it. He wasn't the only one: the poet Guillaume Apollinaire, the playwright Edmond Rostand, the painter Gustav Klimt, and the president of Brazil, Rodrigo Alves, were also victims, not to mention 40 million other people worldwide. The disease took more lives than the battles of World War I. This number seems all the more horrifying now when one takes into account that at the time, the world's population was lower and air travel nonexistent. With today's transportation, the virus would spread with unimaginable speed. Some estimate that it would kill 200 million people.

What has this to do with bird flu? H1N1, the strain behind the ravages of 1918, can be thought of as a younger cousin to H5N1. Could something similar to 1918's crisis with H5N1 happen? Just how closely related are these cousins? Seeking answers to these questions, a team of scientists from the Armed Forces Institute of Pathology went to Alaska in 1997, to a village devastated by the Spanish flu three generations earlier, in order to try to isolate the virus remaining on bodies preserved by the extreme cold.

In their work, the researchers came up against the reluctance of villagers frightened by the idea that exhuming the bodies would cause a new outbreak. The memory of grandparents who'd died from the disease still haunted them. However, the village's council gave the scientists permission to dig, provided that they work without masks to prove there was no danger.

Research began in a small cemetery at the edge of the village. Owing to temperatures under 40 below, it took scientists several days to free the bodies. One of the first was a young woman perfectly preserved thanks to the cold and her corpulence. From her lungs, the team took samples that were immediately sent under high surveillance to labs in the continental United States. A research team led by Robert G. Webster of St. Jude Children's Research Hospital in Memphis, Tennessee, proved that the virus was indeed of the same influenza-causing strain as H5N1, and NS1, a protein violently destructive at a cellular level, was found to be present in both. The NS1 protein is usually only found in typically avian viruses, but the H5N1 and H1N1 strains, capable of infecting humans, are exceptions.

There are other similar examples: Prior to 1918, history had already witnessed avian flu in France. In 1957, the "Asian flu" left 4 million dead, about seventy thousand of them in the United States. The strain to blame in that case was H2N2. In 1968, the H3N2 strain claimed 2 million people in Hong Kong.

In other words, we face a very real threat, for just as in 1918, 1957, and 1968, no vaccine is available. In light of this, the frenzy of precautions and preventive measures all around the world makes more sense. Obviously, there is no known way to stop birds from migrating. As a result, the threat is of great scope.

Science has confirmed that a migrating bird was the source of the Spanish flu that devastated the Alaskan village. The virus can spread even to very cold and hostile regions. Birds cover the entire planet in flight. We are no more protected in the city than in the country, no more on a desert isle than in the desert itself. A wild goose can travel up to 930 miles a day.

Five Billion Vectors for H5N1

You read that right: it is estimated that there are, today, 5 billion migrating birds on this planet. When I say that a single gram of bird droppings can contain millions of infectious particles, you can begin to imagine the seriousness of the threat these birds present. From Africa to Asia, birds roam the globe by the billions and, if contaminated, become veritable viral bombs.

Among migrating species, waterfowl such as wild ducks are especially highly exposed to H5N1. These birds, in landing on a body of water, contaminate it, affecting birds that drink from it. Humans can then come into contact with the virus through dead birds, or through the water itself. Even if not affected, humans can serve as carriers, contaminating birds kept as pets, leading to another epizootic episode. A professor in Hong Kong, Guan Yi, has been reporting on the deaths of many migrating birds around Chinese lakes.

Have we cause to panic and fear the worst? Perhaps not. Pigeons, the most common urban bird, are not very susceptible to H5N1. They pass on other diseases, such as psittacosis—which can cause pneumonia in humans—and salmonellosis, so it's always a good idea to stay away from large flocks. And in truth, the role of migrating birds in spreading the virus remains disputed, as the risk varies depending on the direction of migration. Birds going from

Africa toward Europe are less worrying, as heat and high UV exposure have certain "disinfecting" properties. However, movement from east to west has been confirmed as a source of spread: Russia, Turkey, Romania, and France have been affected by birds migrating from Asia.

The bulk of human contamination is still related to human activities: Infected animals are often transported long distances for commercial operations that are poorly regulated, if at all, as was seen in 2005, when H5N1 arrived in Nigeria via poultry from China. It is therefore of the utmost importance to address the dangers of bird-based contamination as a whole, paying attention to the many other illnesses our feathered friends can carry.

Other Avian Viruses

Aside from H5N1, birds have been the vectors of many other deadly diseases, including the West Nile virus. This potent disease causes high fevers, headaches, violent sweating, and often, throat infections. Red patches sometimes appear on the skin, accompanied by swelling of the glands. Among the frightening complications are meningoencephalitis—inflammation of the brain and its membrane—with general convulsions or decreased consciousness and motor trouble, which can lead to cranial nerve paralysis, coma, and even death.

The virus was first noted in 1937 in Uganda, and reappeared in 1963 in southern France, then in 1996 in

Bucharest, Romania, with seven hundred cases of meningitis. The viral sequence was the same in Romania as in Africa. Therefore, if mosquitoes spread the disease, then birds served as the reservoir hosts. Scientists also established that the West Nile virus was brought to Europe by migratory birds.

This explains why it continues to thrive. In 1999, more than sixty people were infected in New York. Seven died. Since then, the virus has remained present in the United States. Scientists at the Research Institute for Developing Areas even suspect that bird sanctuaries allow for its continued existence.

In 2001, forty-eight patients suffered encephalitis as a result of this virus. At the same time, more than six thousand birds died in seventeen states.

Another disease spread by migratory birds is the Sindbis virus. It causes high fever and skin eruptions. First reported in Cairo in 1952, it showed up again in Sweden and Finland in 1980. Again, we can see the geographical range of its spread. One question often comes up with regard to Sindbis, as it is known to survive only two to three days in the blood of birds: Given that a migration often occurs over several weeks, how is it the virus manages to survive? One hypothesis, put forward by the World Health Organization, suggests that birds keep recontaminating each other throughout the length of their flight, as certain species of ducks are known to be resistant to many viruses, and thereby become asymptomatic carriers.

Now let's take a closer look at how the virus passes from animals to human beings.

Dangerous Liaisons

Avian flu viruses are never passed on to human beings via the alimentary canal, but rather via airways. A chicken, for example, by batting its wings, may set the virus adrift in the atmosphere. If someone happens to be close by, he or she will inhale it into the lungs and become contaminated. In rural areas of China, Vietnam, and Cambodia, it is not rare to see peasants living in close contact with animals. Men, women, children, and even infants often sleep but a few feet away from birds and pigs in a single large room. The stage is set for zoonosis, or infection passed from animals to humans.

All animal species can contaminate us: rats, primates, chickens, pigs, cats, and dogs. Let's take rat fleas for example, which can transmit the bubonic plague (or, more precisely, *icterohemorrhagic leptospirosis*), the rat being an indirect vector in this case. This hemorrhagic fever is well known among sewage workers, who are aware that it takes but a single bite to infect an adult. Dogs and cats transmit rabies. I could fill pages with further examples, especially taking insects into account: Mosquitoes are vectors of a hundred or so viral agents, such as malaria, yellow fever, and dengue, and, as discussed in chapter 3, certain ticks carry Lyme disease.

What can we do to limit the spread of zoonotic diseases? We cannot, with one wave of a magic wand, separate people from animals. The solution lies, first and foremost, in prevention: by limiting contact with certain animals and seriously monitoring their presence on an international scale. This would decrease risks considerably. Just picturing the living conditions, as earlier described, of millions of families in Asia should help us understand the scale of the problem. There is a major difference between such conditions and the strict sanitary standards of livestock farming in developed nations. It is vital that developed nations take up their duties and address such issues, for all the human victims of avian flu (216 at the time of this writing) were infected by direct contact with H5N1-infected animals. These deaths might well have been prevented.

The risk of animal-to-human contamination is quite real, yet it pales beside the even greater danger of human-to-human contamination.

The Specter of a Pandemic

For humans to pass H5N1 directly on to other humans, the virus must first mutate. If it did so, we would be in serious jeopardy. An infected person could contaminate ten others in a few hours, and so on, until we were soon faced with a generalized epidemic, or pandemic. As the virus would not make its presence known right away, we would already be behind the eight ball. Someone contaminated in

Asia could, in a few hours on a plane, reach any location and still show no symptoms. Even temperature sensors in airports, designed to detect persons with fevers, would not catch someone in whom the virus was still incubating. Such a person could go on, in the three days that followed, introduce the virus to entire cities without knowing it. All cities with major airports would be at risk.

For the moment, no such mutation of the H5N1 virus has yet been remarked. Still, H5N1 has slowly begun to transform: From the time of the first deaths from avian flu in 2005, its configuration has been changing toward a form transmissible from human to human, as reported in a December 2005 dispatch from the China Ministry of Health. H5N1 has been found in certain Asian pigs, and pig DNA is 99 percent identical to human DNA. Some pig cells are endowed with receptors for avian viruses, which favors multiple infections, increasing the chances of "recombination," resulting in the creation of a virus with new pathogenic and immunogenic properties. In other words, pigs can supply the missing link the virus needs to complete its mutation toward a form transmissible from person to person. That human viruses are found in pig blood every year when flu season hits seems only to support the possibility, all too easily imagined, of the H5N1 virus combining with the classic influenza virus. The resulting virus would be as easily caught as a more ordinary flu, but the flu vaccine would not prove effective against it, a nightmarish scenario for health authorities and researchers, not to mention those infected.

Fortunately, there are indicators that will alert us to

whether the virus has mutated or not, so that we may take the necessary steps. One such is the H5N1's mortality rate among humans. Today it kills one out of two people. If this ratio should decrease to one in five, it would mean the virus had begun to adapt to human beings. The paradox is that, in becoming less virulent, the virus will become much more dangerous, for in "humanizing" itself, it will spread much more quickly. In the May 2004 issue of *Science*, professor Neil M. Ferguson of the Department of Infectious Disease Epidemiology, at Imperial College London, quantified the statistical risk of a new form appearing. According to his article, it would take six hundred human cases of H5N1 to reach a 50 percent probability of human adaptation.

Other situations would also betray the existence of an adapted virus: for instance, if several members of a single family were infected when only one member was in direct contact with an infected animal. In much the same way, as soon as the first cases of medical personnel contamination appeared, scientists would know the virus had mutated. It would then be essential to isolate the new form of H5N1, determine its characteristics, settle on an effective treatment, and perfect a vaccine.

While they conducted that research, the rest of us would likely be facing a pandemic. According to experts, the question is not whether a pandemic will arise, but when. Panicking will do no good: it is essential to prepare ourselves properly. So much the better, then, to make plans now, as one might for a fire drill.

Stock Up on Canned Food

It's useful to take a look at how our ancestors protected themselves from devastating epidemics, which were very common in the past. Their methods were simple: They built reserves of the bare necessities and went into hiding. When disease fell on the population, they stayed locked inside their homes with enough provisions not to have to venture outside, thus limiting their contact with the outside world and decreasing their risk of infection.

People today have lost their instinct for stockpiling. Yet, think back on the scenes of looted New Orleans supermarkets and department stores in the wake of Hurricane Katrina, when people were shooting at each other over a few canned goods. In the event of a pandemic, food stores will be cleaned out in a matter of hours. Common sense dictates that we start setting aside a variety of foods that will keep for years without risk of spoiling.

Canned fruits, vegetables, meats, and fish are valuable allies when it comes to surviving hard times. Contrary to popular wisdom, their vitamin content is as high as that of fresh products. Many vitamins are very light sensitive. Several days of being on the shelf will cause vegetables to lose vitamin content, but immediate canning keeps nutrients stable.

How much food should you stockpile? The critical phase of any hypothetical pandemic lasts about a month. Stock up enough to ensure a varied menu of lunches and dinners for that period. Here is a sample list:

- salad ingredients (corn, beans, peas): thirty 8-ounce cans
- vegetable soups: thirty 32-ounce cartons
- prepared dishes (heat-and-eat or ready-to-serve): thirty 15-ounce cans
- canned fish (tuna, salmon, sardines, mackerel): thirty 6-oz. cans
- canned meats (pork product, corned beef hash, chili): thirty 8-ounce cans
- vegetables (asparagus, corn, tomatoes, spinach, okra): thirty 15-ounce cans
- canned fruit: thirty 15-ounce cans
- milk, condensed or powdered

Add staples such as grains (rice, pasta), sauces, cereal, cookies, crackers, tea, instant coffee, jam, salt, pepper, bottled water, and oil to this list, and you'll be ready to face a crisis. However, food isn't everything. It will be difficult to stay at home all the time, even during a pandemic. Likely as not you'll have to venture into the world at some point or another, exposing yourself to risk of contamination. Luckily, a simple and helpful measure exists for these forays as well: the face mask.

Protection Against Avian Flu

Though they're not impassable barriers, face masks have proven capable of considerably limiting the risk of viral infection, notably among the young, who are often the most exposed. During the Spanish flu of 1918, most of the victims were under thirty years old. Today we know why: for most of those victims, the epidemic was their first exposure to a deadly virus. In 1878, a virus of the same type had already ravaged the population, leaving survivors partially immunized through prior exposure. People born before 1878 proved much more resistant to the virus.

The same is true for avian viruses. In 1968, a virus similar to H5N1 took almost 4 million lives. The epidemic allowed a significant portion of the world population to become partially immunized to H5N1-type infectious agents. Today, we find ourselves in the same situation as in 1918: those born after the 1968 epidemic have no partial immunity and therefore run a higher risk of infection.

In order to protect yourself, squirrel away a few boxes of masks. These will prove quite useful in case of a pandemic, if only to allow you to venture out to the nearest emergency supply distribution point to secure better masks (which will be in limited supply).

What kind of mask should you buy? Masks are classified by official organizations according to their effectiveness. N95 masks are 95 percent efficient at filtering out particles. N99 masks are 99 percent efficient, and N100 are 100 percent efficient. Price varies by degree of protection offered and wear time. All are made of several layers of different materials to provide effective filtration. A word of caution: it is essential to follow the instructions that come with the mask and to ensure a tight fit to your face. A poor fit along your cheek can negate any protective benefits. In addition, some masks on the market do not offer sufficient protection. These are generally cheaper, and have not been rated. Others, like surgical masks, block infectious emissions coming from the wearer but do not protect the wearer from viruses. Still, they are useful, as they keep infected subjects from contaminating those around them. Washable and reusable masks will soon be available, designed for general public use, but medical professionals entering into close and frequent contact with the virus should still opt for N99 or N100 masks. These are disposable, and should be disposed of with care after use, to prevent yet another source of contamination. The wear time indicated by the manufacturer should also be scrupulously respected— take this into account when calculating how many masks to stockpile.

No preventive arsenal is complete without gloves and disposable protective goggles, as the virus can be transmitted ocularly as well. Let me take a moment to mention that washing your hands still remains an essential act in terms of limiting the spread of the virus.

Those who find these various precautions exaggerated should be reminded that avian influenza is not the only airborne danger we may face in the near future. Other pandemics, like SARS, may also recur. Having the bare necessities at your disposal is like having a first-aid kit. Anxiety over a specific danger is considerably reduced with the knowledge that one has seen to all the basic preparations. One final means of defense remains: antiviral medications.

Antivirals

Just what these drugs do is often not clearly understood by the public. Some confuse them with vaccines, and others with antibiotics. In reality, these drugs are neither able to prevent infection (like vaccines), nor to cure the illness (like antibiotics). So what's the point of antivirals? Quite simply, they allow doctors to greatly slow multiplication of the virus in an infected patient. Thanks to this, symptoms are fewer and complications rare. To use an analogy, we might compare them to the fire retardants used to fight forest fires: they don't keep fires from starting, nor do they douse the flames, but they significantly weaken their progress, greatly helping the firefighters in their work.

The most well-known avian antiviral medication is oseltamivir, sold under the trade name Tamiflu, from Hoffmann-La Roche. It is a neuraminidase inhibitor that works to block the dispersal of new viruses in an organism. It can be deployed as a preventive or a curative, but does not act as a vaccine. As a preventive, a single daily dose is sufficient; its protection vanishes as soon as the subject stops taking the drug. To manage and ameliorate an infection, Tamiflu must be administered within two days of the first symptoms. After two days, the virus will already have spread throughout its new host and the medication will have no effect. This explains its failure in Asia, where it was often prescribed up to a week after the start of an illness. The treatment—for adults, a seventy-five-milligram pill, morning and night—is a five-day cycle. For children, the dose varies by weight, and is available as a syrup.

When correctly used, Tamiflu has proved effective, but there are two major problems. The first stems from the fact that current production rates are too slow to satisfy world demand. This is because the drug is made from star anise, an herb from China. Production of the drug is therefore tied directly to the harvest, with all the limitations that entails. To address the supply shortfall, labs have developed synthetic derivatives that should soon be available on the market.

The second problem arises from the isolation, in two Vietnamese patients, of a strain of H5N1 that is resistant to this medication, as reported in the *New England Journal of Medicine*.* Luckily, another antiviral drug has been developed, Relenza (zanamivir). Tamiflu and Relenza are not available without a prescription, so they cannot be stockpiled by individuals "cleaning out" the shelves of the local drugstore. This turns out to be preferable, as it allows authorities to manage distribution and see to it that sufficient quantities are directed to the populations most at risk

*"Oseltamivir Resistance During Treatment of Influenza A (H5N1) Infection," *New England Journal of Medicine* (December 22, 2005): 2667–72.

in case of pandemics: policemen, firemen, and medical and military personnel.

What About Vaccines?

To be absolutely clear: No vaccine that will prevent an avian flu pandemic is currently available. The flu shots we're urged to get every year offer no protection against H5N1. There is only one advantage to getting a flu shot where avian flu is concerned: The onset of any flulike symptoms will, as a result, be ascribed to avian flu and not a more ordinary strain of influenza, allowing the appropriate measures to be taken more quickly. Another vaccine of interest in this context, especially with the elderly or immune deficient, is the antipneumococcal vaccine. The H5N1 virus is a source of many complications, notably a secondary pulmonary infection by pneumococcus, which this vaccine can help contain.

As I have said, we must await the first cases of interhuman infection before a vaccine can be developed specifically for the H5N1 virus and produced on an industrial scale. This process may take up to six months, during which a pandemic will rage. New technologies using cell lines are being studied, with a view to shortening the latency period and augmenting production capacities. The difficulty is that the virus's exact signature must be known in order to produce a vaccine: it's no use making a key without knowing what the lock looks like. The World Health

Organization recommends preparing other vaccines using recently isolated strains.

With the January 2007 H5N1 outbreaks in Hungary, health authorities launched a campaign to vaccinate the entire populace. However, the vaccine used had not received the endorsement of worldwide scientific authorities, which raised the question of its actual effectiveness and health risks. In any case, this episode brought fears of avian flu to the fore once again, as was shown in the decisions of neighboring countries to place an immediate ban on the importation of poultry from Hungary, while all affected livestock were slaughtered. It remains difficult, despite drastic sanitary measures, to completely eliminate the risk that live, contaminated game and fowl will reach the market.

Running A-Fowl

Chickens, ducks, and geese, unlike humans, can be immunized. Programs that do so have been in place since 2005 in China, especially in sensitive regions. In the meantime, as this task is carried out, is it safe to consume fowl? The answer is simple: yes. Effective systems are in place to insure our safety. A first fundamental point is that chickens are sold plucked and gutted. Whole plucked chickens are risk-free. Handling an unplucked and infected chicken carries with it the risk of infection from inhaling particles of dried droppings in the feathers.

Again, the H5N1 virus cannot be contracted via alimentary transmission, so consuming an infected animal is not an issue. Even if you should ingest contaminated meat, there is little chance that H5N1 will survive in your stomach: gastric juices will destroy it, however slowly. Ten seconds of cooking at 140 degrees Fahrenheit are enough to reduce viral presence by a factor of ten, and at 150 degrees by a factor of one hundred. At 160 degrees, no trace of the virus remains. Muscle should be cooked through thoroughly: this means that white meat must be white, not pink. The virus resists freezing, but on the other hand is sensitive to salt as well as ultraviolet light.

Nor should you avoid eggs, so long as they too are properly prepared. A sick bird normally stops laying, which already reduces your chance of finding contaminated eggs on the market. However, it's possible for infected poultry to lay eggs during the virus's incubation period, in which case the white, yolk, or shell may contain the virus. Once more, thorough cooking quickly kills off the virus. At the time of this writing there is no epidemiological evidence that avian flu can be contracted by consuming the eggs of any sick or healthy bird, whether its eggs are fully cooked or not.

Turbulent Times Ahead

Flu outbreaks tend to be cyclical. At the time of this writing, in the early 2000s, the world is entering a period during which avian flu regularly makes headlines (as it did in the first half of 2006) and then subsides from view (as it did in the second half of 2006, when nothing of note really happened and we told ourselves we'd gotten all worked up over nothing), before rearing its awful head again, as it did in the first three months of 2007.

We're in for a bumpy ride.

We know that avian flu has killed 216 people and that the threat of a pandemic looms large, but we don't know when it will strike. Public health agencies must respond to every cry of wolf without letting their guard down even once. Making the most of these periods of relative calm by continuing to search for breakthroughs in production methods for vaccines will help maximize our chances of containing a pandemic when the alarm sounds.

Cats: High-Risk Pets?

Hygiene is in fashion, germs are on the run. And the ASPCA isn't lifting a finger to help them.
—Alphonse Allais

Cats have been the privileged companions of human beings for millennia, but their unanimously appreciated grace and sociability aren't without drawbacks. In addition to provoking allergies, cats can spread disease: toxoplasmosis, pasteurellosis, cat scratch fever, and more recently even avian flu, which has been decidedly rampant for some time. But are these animals really a danger to humans?

A Succession of Remarkable Occurrences

The first indications of a link between cats and bird flu appeared in 2004 in the Netherlands. A team in Rotterdam led by the professor and veterinarian Albert Osterhaus conducted tests showing that cats experimentally infected with H5N1 died quickly. Moreover, the virus could be found in feline excretions and nasal secretions. A host of different events followed: In January 2006, an infected kitten was isolated living near affected livestock. In February, at a home in Nakornpathom, Thailand containing fifteen cats, three tested positive for H5N1. In the end, fourteen died. On February 28, 2006, a cat carrying the virus was found dead on the German island of Rügen. A few days later, papers mentioned the death of a cat that had consumed the carcass of a diseased pigeon. Finally, on March 6, 2006, three pet cats were identified as H5N1 carriers in Graz, Austria.

These troubling discoveries over a short period of time cast suspicion on the possible transmissibility of the disease from cats to people. The worry has been that if a large number of cats contract H5N1, they might provide the vehicle for mutation to a strain that could lead to an epidemic among humans. More research is urged by Dr. Osterhaus.

No Proven Contamination

Cats appear to be epidemiological dead ends for the virus: Affected felines excrete very little virus. In fact, a cat's genetic environment is unfavorable to the multiplication of H5N1, which is good news. Practically speaking, an affected subject has very little chance of infecting one of its fellow creatures or members of another species. For example, the cat that died in Rügen was probably infected by inhaling viral particles from the feathers or droppings of a bird who died of H5N1. However, the Dutch study already cited shows that it is experimentally possible to infect cats by feeding them day-old H5N1-infected chicks, and introduces the notion of possible cat-to-cat transmission. Moreover, the work of Dr. Roongroje Thanawongnuwech, a veterinary pathologist in Thailand, established the existence of H5N1 transmission from tiger to tiger. Leopards have also been infected in a Thai zoo. The feline family seems to display a certain weakness toward the virus, but one thing is for certain: to this day, there has been no case anywhere in the world of a human being infected by a cat or other member of the *Felidae* family.

For all that, events are still too recent to give us a full picture: The infection of cats by the H5N1 virus in 2006 is a first in Europe. The possibility of mutation in the cat, along with the fact that cats can be infected via the digestive tract and sporadically excrete the virus, are cause for concern.

Whatever the truth turns out to be, stray cats should not in any way be considered simple cuddly creatures on which to shower our affections, since it is known for certain that cats can transmit other diseases, starting with the one known as "cat scratch fever."

Germs with Their Claws Out

There is a renewed outbreak of this complaint every year between August and January, with an incidence of about one case for every ten thousand people. This may seem insignificant, but the statistic is misleading, as many of the ten thousand people are not cat owners. The proportion of affected subjects among cat owners is much higher.

Cat scratch fever usually involves animals infected by a gram-negative bacillus called *Bartonella henselae*. Cats can pass this on to humans by scratching, biting, or through the intermediary vectors of fleas. Symptoms include glandular swelling, often around the neck or armpits. This lasts for several months, sometimes evolving into suppuration, or pus discharge. In other cases, a complication known as Parinaud's oculoglandular syndrome develops, combining conjunctivitis with glandular swelling near the ear. Much less frequently, neurological problems (encephalitis), hepatitis, and bone infection (osteomyelitis) have been recorded, especially among children. Finally, subjects with cardiac valve prostheses or valve difficulties have contracted valvular infections caused by *Bartonella henselae*, some of which have required surgical intervention and valve replacement.

Blood tests can confirm diagnosis; the treatment is a course of antibiotics. No real preventive measure exists for this illness other than avoiding the company of cats. A good habit for cat owners to adopt is consulting their physicians in case of any suspicious swelling of the glands.

Pasteurellosis

This pathology has several things in common with cat scratch fever, starting with its cause: a gram-negative bacillus, known in this case as *Pasteurella multocida*. Contamination still proceeds from bites or scratches, but there the resemblance ends. The first difference is that dogs are also vectors of this disease, although much more rarely so. Second, the incubation period is very short—often just a few hours after transmission. A third difference concerns the manifestation of the disease: among the parts of the body, hands are the most often affected and will be seized with great pain. The area around the scratch or bite will swell noticeably and bleed freely. There are sometimes complications with acute inflammation (phlegmon), swelling of the axillary glands, or arthritis. It is therefore important to consult your practicing physician quickly after a scratch or bite that seems to be taking a turn for the worse. He or she will able to prescribe an antibiotic treatment that will take care of pasteurellosis in a few days.

Toxoplasmosis

This pathology is much more common and affects a small percentage of pregnant women as well, for whom it can prove quite dangerous, as it significantly raises the risk of miscarriage. The fetus may suffer a number of disorders such as hemorrhaging, fever, or encephalopathy, which are often fatal. If not, disease can still attack the fetus's eyes, causing blindness, or cause psychomotor difficulties, convulsions, and hydrocephaly to appear several years after birth.

In short, this pathology is not to be ignored. Know, first of all, that contamination generally occurs via the consumption of foods soiled by cat feces containing infectious organisms known as oocysts, the source of the disease. It may be hard to imagine that foods can be contaminated in this manner, but all it takes is a cat jumping on the table and getting close to food. Most of the time, no one even notices, as cats are usually quiet and agile. Fruits and vegetables may have been contaminated prior to their purchase. In addition to the cat vector, contamination by ingestion of insufficiently cooked meat is also possible.

Once the disease is full-blown, glandular swelling may be noted up and down the neck. The subject will often complain of unexplained fatigue. A blood test will confirm the diagnosis and antibiotics can be prescribed for rapid recovery. As mentioned earlier, some women contract the disease at a young age and become naturally immunized. But be careful: if this not the case, expectant mothers are strictly advised to avoid all contact with cats, in order to avoid any tragedy, even if it means lodging their own pets with friends for nine months. In addition, very young children and patients undergoing chemotherapy should not handle the litter box. Fruits and vegetables should always be well washed, meats thoroughly cooked, and raw meats avoided.

Not All Immune Systems
Are Created Equal

Microbes have no time to study biologists.
—HENRI MICHAUX

According to the World Health Organization, thirty new diseases for which neither vaccines nor curative treatments exist have emerged in the past twenty years. Today, we're engaged in a race against the clock and must confront new viruses spreading ever more rapidly around the world. Avian flu might worry us quite justly right now, but tomorrow ever more formidable microbial agents could appear. In short, the risk of a pandemic is higher now than ever before. What are some of the reasons for this?

Varied Vulnerabilities

A century ago, Pasteur was already saying, "Germs are nothing. Their environment is everything." In other words, the same infectious agent does not act with the same intensity on two different people. Some hosts prove to be much more vulnerable than others. Herein lies one of the first reasons for the emergence of so many new diseases: over the past twenty years, the fastest-growing groups have happened to be the most vulnerable—including the elderly, as scientific advances extend our life-span and the baby boom generation comes of age. But the older we get, the weaker our immune systems get; an ordinary flu can be fatal for a ninety-year-old. This is why flu shots are recommended for the elderly. Senior citizens are not the only group with higher susceptibility to infectious diseases: people undergoing chemotherapy or corticosteroid treatments; transplant recipients; and people with AIDS, diabetes, or other serious chronic immunodeficiency conditions provide first targets for microbial agents. Their ranks are also increasing as medicine manages to keep them alive longer than before.

The genetic makeup of individuals is also greatly responsible for variations in susceptibility. Some variations possess a natural immunity to various viruses, including even HIV. On the other hand, others carry a gene that makes them susceptible to salmonella, for example.

More People, More Travel, More Viruses

The rising number of subjects susceptible to viruses does not explain everything: the considerable growth in world population in the past few years also plays an undeniable part. Population density in certain areas of the world has reached an extreme; the danger of infection skyrockets with overcrowding, especially when entire families share a room with livestock—which is, as I've mentioned, often the case in Asia. Such situations promote zoonosis, the depredations of which I've discussed in previous sections.

What's more, these runaway demographics coincide with the end of a certain kind of isolation among global populations. With modern air travel, the inhabitants of a Chinese farm are no more than a half day away from most major cities. Imagine this all-too-likely scenario: One day a farmer living in close contact with his animals is unknowingly contaminated. He goes to the market in a neighboring village to sell his wares. There, he contaminates a wholesaler, who takes a plane bound for Los Angeles a few hours later. After almost a day's flight, he passes through U.S. customs without the slightest trace of illness. But as soon as the incubation period is up, he is in danger of passing his germs on to dozens of people he meets in the street.

Other elements have a role in the rise of disease as well, such as massive deforestation. This has resulted in humans and certain animals coming into an unnatural contact that would never have come about had it not been for human intrusion, as these animals are proven carriers of infectious diseases for which our immune systems are unprepared.

Changes in climate are also a factor. Even without the natural disasters brought about in every corner of the world as a result, global warming as we know it—for it is happening all around us—has a significant impact. With the rise in temperature, certain vectors of microbial agents that previously existed only in tropical climates will soon find broader areas favorable to their development. Here again, our immune defenses are forced to confront new pathogenic agents for which they are not necessarily adapted.

Ethics and Responsibility

Experience with epidemics and natural disasters enables society to anticipate the catastrophic consequences of a pandemic on personal, public, and social life, as well as the risk of violence that may result. Faced with this state of affairs, it is crucial for public health administrators, institutions, and corporations to include notions of ethics, transparency, and integrity into the steps taken toward prevention, and to make provision for irrational behavior. Corporations, especially, must take responsibility for their actions.

Natural Immunity

The presence of all the new dangers discussed here can seem quite disheartening, leaving little reason for optimism. But while these threats are many and quite real, it's better by far to fight the natural urge to deny them, and instead study them with lucidity, in order to be ready to confront them. Prevention, information, and the rules of hygiene are the trump cards in this game.

Throughout its history, humanity has had many run-ins with catastrophic diseases, and has always come through.

The key idea has been to avoid contact with the virus as much as possible by living off stockpiled goods, and also by employing practical, specific methods to drive away viruses and bacteria, or at least their carriers. In 1630, during the plague, some inhabitants of Milan never left their homes without a pistol to ward off anyone who drew too close. In 1720, authorities in Marseille decided to build a wall around the city to limit the risk of certain diseases. Fortunately, everything is easier today: vaccines and face masks constitute very effective protection against the spread of disease.

Humanity has always had among its ranks individuals whose constitutions have enabled them to survive epidemics. Even faced with the most savage pathogenic agents, such as leprosy, tuberculosis, or the plague, a portion of the population has proved resistant. These survivors have come through different scourges that have decimated the planet's population, thanks to inherently superior immune defenses. In a certain way, we are all descendants of the fittest among our predecessors, hence the question: Do people who are naturally immune to these new pathogens exist today?

The example of AIDS has brought a positive response to this inquiry, according to an article in the August 1996 issue of *Cell*. A team of American scientists studied the genetic makeup of two men who, although frequent sexual partners of people who were HIV-positive, had remained completely negative in the absence of all protection. Both men had something in common: dual mutations in the

CKR-5 gene, a coreceptor necessary for the AIDS virus to penetrate a cell. Without this coreceptor, the virus cannot target and invade cells, and thus remains harmless. By virtue of the mutation, these men possessed a sort of natural genetic armor protecting them from the virus.

Along the same lines, Duncan and Scott of the University of Liverpool found that people with a genetic mutation of the type CCR5-△32 are protected from AIDS even after having contracted HIV, as this mutation keeps the virus from destroying the immune system. According to their studies, a proportional increase in people with CCR5-△32 resulted from the plague in Europe, as a number of survivors from that era were carriers of the mutation. Duncan and Scott estimate that 10 percent of Europeans share this peculiarity, adding that in Scandinavian countries ravaged by the plague in Copenhagen in 1711, the rate of resistance was as high as 15 percent of the population. Such information in no way advocates going without a condom, but it does show that even when faced with dangers of great magnitude, like AIDS, humanity is far from being without hope.

There are hard times ahead, in which such inherent capacities for resistance will prove valuable, just as valuable as the rules of hygiene, which themselves form the first line of defense against disease.

A Final Word

Hygiene, like manners, reflects the attitudes of entire societies. The rules of hygiene change from century to century and country to country, with each culture and religion, adapting, evolving. Today, we stand on a cusp between ancient superstition and scientific and technological progress. As a result, certain hygienic habits have proved their usefulness and contribute in a real way to our health and well-being. Others reveal themselves to be much less helpful, being closer to rituals and tribal or religious customs than they are to verified preventive measures.

Today, with efficient tools at our disposal, we have a unique opportunity, unprecedented in human history, to evaluate the precise effectiveness of each preventive measure. We are aware that from now on, our health will be more and more in our own hands. We can change the course of history by practicing habits that we know will protect us, ridding ourselves of those no longer useful, and enjoying new-found freedom from antiquated superstitions.

Good hygiene—the first line of medical defense—lies within the reach of each and every one of us.